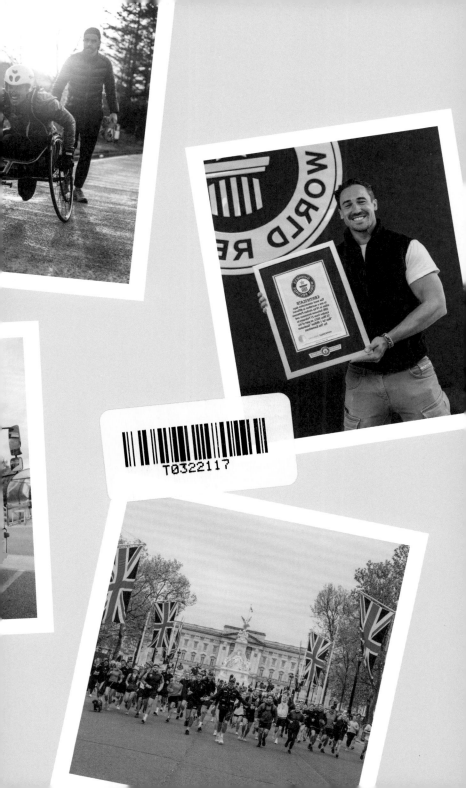

T0322117

Fortune Favours the Brave

Fortune Favours the Brave

76 Short Lessons on
Finding Strength in Vulnerability

JOSHUA PATTERSON

PENGUIN LIFE

AN IMPRINT OF

PENGUIN BOOKS

PENGUIN LIFE

UK | USA | Canada | Ireland | Australia
India | New Zealand | South Africa

Penguin Life is part of the Penguin Random House group of companies
whose addresses can be found at global.penguinrandomhouse.com.

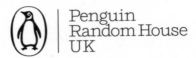

Penguin
Random House
UK

First published 2024

001

Copyright © Joshua Patterson, 2024

The moral right of the author has been asserted

Set in 13.5/16pt Garamond MT Std
Typeset by Jouve (UK), Milton Keynes
Printed and bound in Great Britain by Clays Ltd, Elcograf S.p.A.

The authorized representative in the EEA is Penguin Random House Ireland,
Morrison Chambers, 32 Nassau Street, Dublin D02 YH68

A CIP catalogue record for this book is available from the British Library

ISBN: 978-0-241-68254-8

www.greenpenguin.co.uk

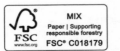

For India, and my family

Introduction

When I was asked to write this book, I had just finished running 76 marathons in 76 days to raise money for the Samaritans. I was a world record holder, and the publisher thought the lessons I had learned during this challenge would make a great book. And they would have done. But once I began thinking about writing it, I realized that being able to complete the challenge was the *result* of all the lessons I had learned in the years before. It was the outcome, not the journey. My 42-kilometre runs around every city in the United Kingdom happened because of the changes I had made earlier in my life, and this book is a collection of the simple lessons I learned along the way.

I wanted to support the Samaritans because there was a time in my twenties when I couldn't think of a single reason to keep on living. I am very open about my previous struggles with my mental health because I want to normalize them. Coming out of my battles with mental illness, it felt like I had been given a second chance at life. Knowing that the Samaritans provided support in all 76 cities in the UK, it made complete sense for me to run a marathon in each one to raise awareness around their work and the rise of mental illness.

This isn't a book about how to run 3,207 kilometres in two and a half months. It's not about record-breaking, endurance tests or extreme sports. It's not even really about running.

While doing this latest challenge, runners kept asking me about performance metrics – the focus mainly being on the speed at which I ran. But do you know what? I didn't care about my speed or marathon timings. It felt so irrelevant to what I was trying to achieve. This wasn't about speed. It was about connection. All I cared about was waking up, eating breakfast, and stepping onto that starting line, regardless of the pain I was in. I knew that when we set off at 9 a.m., we would finish at around 3.30 p.m., sometimes later, depending on who was running with me or how I felt that day. It wasn't about the technicalities of how I completed a feat that no one else had ever achieved. For me, it was much more about experiencing the journey. Technicalities would never have helped me anyway, because by the end, my body was slowly breaking down due to several injuries, and at that point it was all about mind over matter.

Sometimes, the science behind how we do these things gets in the way. The beauty of the lessons I've learned from the people around me and the situations I've been in is how much you can achieve when you don't get caught up in the details, and just decide to start something new. Instead of having tunnel vision, take a minute and look around you. Maybe you too can take inspiration from the people in your life or what you've been through in the past.

So, rather than being about marathons, this book is about empathy. We all face difficult times throughout our lives. Although we struggle in different ways, we're all connected by the struggle. For me, it's about identifying the personal hurdles we each face and how we can potentially make somebody else's journey easier for them.

The beginning of this process started six years ago, when one of my best friends, Tano, was in a serious motorbike accident in which he could have died. Having battled suicidal thoughts in the past and been close to taking my own life, I identified with the challenge Tano was facing even though the adversity was different. He had lost the use of his legs, but equally he was still alive and had a second chance at life. It made me think about what I'd done to get through the dark point I had faced, and how I could try to convert that period of recovery into something relatable to him. I hoped to help him, so that he could then pass that on to someone else down the line.

Although I have had struggles in my life, many people face much tougher times and don't have access to the resources I have, so this is something I knew I wanted to help with. I have committed my life to ensuring I can help as many of those people in need as possible. Helping Tano was the beginning of a chain reaction of individual journeys that would change lives. There is a formula here that hundreds of people have already used, and it works. The simplicity is what makes it so successful. By striving to achieve something, you will in turn inspire others to do the same, so that we can all support ourselves to find strength in places we didn't know we had it, and live fulfilled lives.

This isn't a book solely for those who have been through the extreme circumstances of life-and-death situations or near-fatal accidents. What you have faced and the changes you want to make might be very different. You might just feel that something isn't quite right in your life or that you lack purpose, and that the solution might relate to art, creativity or a new career, rather than exercise. Your aspirations or goals will also change during your life as you accomplish more and more. As soon as I finished setting this world record, people kept on asking, 'What's next?'

What's next is this book. A completely different type of achievement, but one that is particularly challenging for me. Because of how my brain works, writing a book is a huge hurdle, but I wanted to do it because it takes me out of my comfort zone.

That's why it is written slightly differently from others you might have read recently. The chapters are intentionally short because I know that an ADHD mind like mine, or a preoccupied mind, might struggle to focus on longer ones. My brain runs at 100 miles an hour, and I need a simpler structure for things to sink in. I also know that anyone with a cluttered mind needs something that's easy to interact with, and many of us have these busy brains if we're going through mental health or life struggles. I don't want the potential solutions to be more difficult to absorb than they need to be.

I hope that this book offers you a fresh approach to life. It includes 76 simple lessons that I have learned on how to achieve your goals while accepting your whole self. It's about how to find the lightness in the dark times, and how to use every experience to your advantage. Mental health can have a weight to it, so let's not load you up with another burden or responsibility. I want you to approach this book however you want. Read the entire thing from start to finish, or dip in and out if you feel that's best for you. I'd suggest you read the first few chapters, as they lay the foundations, but after that, carry on through the rest of the book or jump around. Use the lessons I have learned in whichever way you want and need at the time.

What I'm trying to do is create something universal, that's open to anybody and helpful to everyone – whether it's with mental health, physical health, confidence, or even work problems. Whatever you feel might be holding you back, or whatever you want to aim for, there will be something in this book to help you.

The real challenge for me is executing this book and doing it well. And if this book is my current hurdle, I hope as you read it you'll start thinking about what your own is and, by the end, have some tools for how to leap over it. What has kept me going in creating this book is imagining it in someone's home, where they read it themselves and find a reason to do something that changes their life in some way – or even gift it to someone else or pass on the advice. That is a motivating thing to envisage.

Whether you are at a low point right now or not, there is always more to explore, experience and create. So let's start at the beginning – all about how to rise again.

Lesson 1: Rise Like a Phoenix

When I got the call back in 2017 that one of my best friends, Tano, had been in a motorbike accident and was paralysed from the waist down, my life took a different direction. I found a new purpose. The immediate concern was to support Tano through his recovery, but around a year later, when he was using a wheelchair, that rippled out to taking on challenges to raise awareness and money for charities that I am passionate about.

What is so inspiring about Tano is that he is confident in himself and proud of what others might see as a vulnerability. Yes, he was in a wheelchair for a long time and had a life-changing disability, but that was never what you focused on when you met him then. He has always radiated positive energy that others are drawn to. He put hard work, determination and that positive energy into his recovery, and how he handled his situation taught me so much about how to approach life.

A couple of years later, in 2019, I was in the middle of setting a new world record for travelling from John O'Groats to Land's End by wheelchair. It was brutal. Nineteen days of hell covering 950 miles, when the furthest I'd gone in a wheelchair before the challenge was 30 miles. The gradients I faced were double what I had done before – Scotland is no stranger to a hill – and I only had my arms to power me up those steep inclines. By the second day, my hands were covered in weeping blisters, and my stomach and back muscles were spasming. I knew from then on I would just have to tackle it one hill at a time.

I faced sheer inclines day after day. At times my progression was so slow that George, the challenge pacer, would have to stop cycling and push his bike behind me. We would count fifteen turns of my wheels and then have a few minutes' break. For most people who don't use a wheelchair, their upper-body strength doesn't match their lower-body strength. Turning those wheels with only my arm and chest muscles to propel me forward was so humbling.

Whenever I was struggling, I would say to George, 'Cruise like a tortoise. Rise like a phoenix.' It started as a joke, with George and I occasionally adding a gentle 'Cacaw!' to signal the phoenix being nearby. But after a while, it became a sort of sub-identity. This attitude of rising from the ashes gave so much energy to the team.

The spirit of the phoenix has been a psychological tool I have used in the years since, and is what helped get me through the longest challenge I faced, which was running 76 marathons in 76 days. At times, it felt like I had to morph into the phoenix just to keep putting one foot in front of the other. Spotting one of the team out of the corner of my eye and making a subtle flapping-wing motion would raise a smile and let each of us know we would get through this.

It doesn't matter who you are or what your background is, we all face adversity at some stage. Whether it's a physical disability, material or emotional hardships, or mental illness, there will be tough times. So many people are struggling in some capacity and are on their knees right now. You might be one of them, and I hope this book will help you feel ready to rise again – and help you achieve that.

The image of the phoenix rising again is so fitting for what we face in life, sometimes multiple times. We can return from our lows if we don't let them hold us down. We can find strength in our vulnerability. It is all about rising and reinvigorating, because as long as we're still here, we've got a second chance at life. There is always a different solution to the ones we've tried before, and we all have the ability to set ourselves on a different path and embark on a more positive journey. What's done is done, but tomorrow is a new day.

A phoenix's life is not perfect, and it might need to rise again and again. But after doing it once, we know what is possible. I still have anxiety every day, but I've learned how to cope with it and know how to make improvements. John O'Groats to Land's End showed me that even when we face adversity every day, if we keep pushing forward and have the right people around us, things will always get better.

Everyone has the power to impact the world by changing at least one life within it, starting with their own.

Lesson 2: Find Your Why

It was minus-six degrees outside but it felt like minus-fourteen inside the camper van. Our home for eleven weeks while I completed the Run41Million challenge – 76 marathons in 76 days around the 76 cities in the UK – didn't give us as much protection from the cold as we had hoped for, which didn't make for the best night's sleep. It was early morning, and I had to leave soon to run the next marathon, in Sunderland. Someone was knocking on the door to my part of the camper van, but I didn't want to get up. The day before, I had run my sixteenth consecutive marathon, in Newcastle, where I'd spent the last few kilometres running in the snow.

I rolled over and away from the sound of knocking. My Achilles tendon, which had been playing up over the last little while, let me know it still wasn't anywhere near healed. I had damaged it a few days before, nearly ending the challenge.

I wondered why I was doing this to myself – why I did any of these things to myself. Then I thought about the people I could help, the charities I supported and the work they were doing. The knocking at my door started up again. Sighing, I threw off the fourteen blankets I was huddled underneath and let my videographer and wingman, Reece, into my small room. I had another marathon to run.

Understanding your 'Why' in life is a crucial ingredient in moving forward, and it reminds you to look to the past and then the future. Ask yourself *why* you are at this point in your life. Then ask yourself *why* you want to make a change. You might have gotten to the point where you're tired of feeling like shit, or sick of not progressing, or being constantly on your knees, or staying in a destructive relationship. There can be so many reasons. Once you know what your reason is and can name it, you are using the reality of your situation to propel you forward. That's when your journey begins.

Your Why is also about what motivates you and gives you purpose. Not everyone knows their purpose, and there is the real risk of going through life and never finding it. For me, my Why is gratitude for a second chance at life. In my darkest time I almost lost my life to suicide, which is covered later in this book, and I really want to commit to that second chance in the best possible way. I want to use that gift to help people from all walks of life, no matter what adversity they face, and use my journey to help them progress.

Finding your Why is about finding your purpose. It doesn't have to be running, completing challenges or even anything physical. It could be a new career, reading more, finding inspiration as an artist again or even playing tiddlywinks. Purpose looks different for every individual, and success is relative.

My gratitude for a second chance at life has made me want to help other people. I found myself in a wheelchair travelling the length of the UK because one of my best friends was paralysed from the waist down. I then found myself out of the wheelchair and running, because my body was being damaged by the challenges I was doing in it. The way the Why journey is put into practice can be unpredictable, but also exciting, because you don't know where it's going to take you.

Ultimately, it's about discovering what you're meant to do and finding the strength to do it. It doesn't really matter what your purpose is – we all find our inspiration in different ways and it comes from different things (thankfully, or it would be a very bland world we live in).

All through this journey and these challenges I have used my gratitude for life to keep me motivated and to shift my mindset away from the negatives of a situation towards the positives. When I hear about what other people have been through in their lives, and the people they might have lost, it makes me grateful for my own life and I use this gratitude to help others. This mindset is similar to running a marathon – just putting one foot in front of the other. I've become persistent. I've learned resilience. I was born and built exactly the same as everyone else. But it's the mindset I have developed that enables me to do these things and not give up.

There were times during the 76 Marathons that I would wake up in the morning and couldn't even contemplate setting my foot on that start line because of the state I was in. Somehow I still managed to run an entire marathon every time. Was that because I'm exceptional? I don't think so. It was because the Why behind what I was doing was so powerful that it overtook everything else I was feeling.

You might not know your Why straight away. It may take time to come to you, and is often about being open to new experiences and the signs nudging you along. The way in which I decided to fulfil my Why has changed over the years, and that wouldn't have happened if I wasn't open to other possibilities. And for me, the process all began with a flatmate who wouldn't accept that I didn't like running.

Lesson 3: Try New Things

It was 6 a.m., and my flatmate JoJo's bright, beaming face peered around my bedroom door. He had woken me up to ask if I wanted to run 5 kilometres with him. I thought about ducking out but knew my body needed some exercise, so I reluctantly pulled myself out of bed.

As we pounded the streets together, my throat started tightening up. There was a burning sensation in my chest telling me that my lungs weren't getting enough air, even though I was panting. JoJo was ahead, effortlessly gliding along like some sort of gazelle, not even breaking out in a sweat. My pride wouldn't let me drop too far back, so I was gasping behind him. Everything ached, and I was already exhausted. I bloody hated running.

That was just three years ago, and I still say that I'm not a great runner. Even when I first started training for the challenge of 76 marathons in 76 days, the furthest I'd ever run was 10 kilometres, which is just under a quarter of a marathon. I had a long way to go. But that was the reason I decided to begin these running challenges. It was precisely because I hated running that I knew it would be a test of my mindset.

It took a long time for me to fall in love with running, and it didn't happen until I first tasted trail running in

Spain. Running made complete sense to me when I was out in the countryside. Beautiful views surrounded me, with different elevations and terrain to keep my mind engaged. I didn't even know that it was called 'trail running' at the time. I just thought I was training with an ex-SAS guy by running around a mountain. It wasn't until later that I realized how spending time outdoors can have a huge impact on our mental health, and therefore our resilience when it comes to doing hard things.

Running is also something that most people, in theory, can get involved with. When I did my 76 Marathons challenge, I wanted to see as many people as possible join me on each marathon, even if it meant they only came along for a short time. I thought that's something most people could achieve, and I wanted to make the challenge as accessible as I could.

When I began training for the 76 Marathons, I realized there was already a huge network of established ultra-runners. There are a lot of people in the ultra-marathon space who have done mind-boggling distances in the most inhospitable conditions. All those individuals are godlike in their endurance and have put years into training and perfecting their technique, whereas I would always be the nincompoop on the sidelines just giving it a go. At the age of thirty-one years old, I was a complete novice but I still wanted to join in on the fun. And why not?

To be honest, I'm just as surprised as the next person that I found myself doing these challenges, because for a while I didn't really understand how I could complete these endurance tests. I'm not coming from a scientific background. I'm not a Gurkha or Special Forces. I'm just a regular person who had a bit of a shit life at times and decided to do some crazy things. But if I'd looked at this ultra-marathon space and thought, 'That's not for a person like me,' I wouldn't be where I am now.

Like how school teaches us one approach to education, often there seems to be only one blueprint for life, and you're expected to follow it. And if you don't want to, you fall behind. We need to start tearing up the blueprint and going out and trying new things. Things we might be rubbish at or where it's expected that people look a certain way, or things that are taken super seriously and we can bring a bit of a new energy to them.

When you look at people 'up there' who have done extraordinary things, remember that they all started as beginners too. A lack of experience didn't stop them from trying out new things. There's also no need to put any pressure on yourself, because all you're doing at this stage is trying something new. You don't need to be the best — you just need to make a start.

Lesson 4: Surround Yourself with the Right People

Around a year after Tano's accident, I found myself in Richmond Park learning how to use a wheelchair. I'd spent the previous year by Tano's side during his recovery, and he had asked me to do the Berlin Marathon with him – both of us in wheelchairs. I said yes despite not knowing how to use a wheelchair and certainly not knowing how to race 42 kilometres in one. Hence the need for the Weir Archer Academy in Richmond to show me the wheelchair ropes.

A camera crew were filming us to make a documentary about Tano's accident and recovery. The idea was that this marathon was a way of me helping my friend find his legs once again. The irony was that, as those cameras started rolling, the bottom fell out of my own world in three different ways – bad things really do come in threes. I was in bits as I was hit time and again with life-changing situations and news over the course of a few months. This documentary, which was supposed to be about me helping my friend in need, ended up with a complete role reversal as he helped me through one of my darkest times.

I was knocked sideways, and for six months I found myself in such a rut that I didn't want to even get out of bed. The last thing I wanted to do was train for a marathon; in fact it felt like the wrong time to set myself any kind of challenge. But I had made a promise to Tano, and he needed this as part of his recovery journey. I had also learned in recent years that, despite what I was feeling, I wouldn't let myself succumb to those negative emotions. So, every day I made myself go to the park in my wheelchair simply because it gave me a reason to wake up and leave the house. Sometimes when something is perceived as a hindrance, it's actually a saviour.

Looking back, the whole situation was actually my saving grace. My best friend got me through one of the worst times in my life by giving me a purpose and supporting me with his friendship when I needed it most. We laugh about this now – how quickly our roles reversed when I needed him.

Since then, I have tried to surround myself with exceptional people, as I know they play such an important role in the outcome of a person's life. You might not have found that group or those individuals yet, and that's okay. It took me a while to find mine as well. It was through discovering my purpose and Why over the years that led me to them. The great thing about finding a new challenge, purpose or goal is that it also opens you up to a new community. Running groups or clubs are a classic example of this. They're usually really genuine groups who welcome newcomers and are filled with people of all ages and backgrounds. Wherever your purpose lies, it is likely there is a similar ready-built community of people who you will automatically have something in common with.

There are so many ways in which the people around you can be exceptional. They might have an infectious personality, or be loving, empathetic, creative or dedicated. Despite never having run a marathon before, Simon, my biokinetics coach, decided to join me on my Run 4 Nations challenge to run a marathon in each country in the UK in twenty-four hours – and, although it wasn't easy, he did it. Later, when I messaged him on a morning during the 76 Marathons challenge, complaining about it raining, he simply said, 'Lions don't get bothered by the rain,' and that set me up for the day. He had taken the time to remind me that I could do this. Simon's dedication was exceptional, and that, in turn, helped to spur me on and reminded me that I could do hard things.

What makes people special is unique to them, but what unites them is their positive energy. When you find these people whose presence lifts you up, hold them close. You might not know when you will next need a bit of extra help but, when you do, they're the sort of people who are happy to roll up their sleeves and do some of the heavier lifting.

Lesson 5:
Don't Listen to the Doubters

One of the best perks about running 76 marathons in 76 days was the number of people I was able to chat to as we jogged through city streets and along countryside lanes. As the challenge progressed, more and more people heard about it and came to join us. I'd often be lost in my head, trying to ignore the pain in my foot, when someone would begin to run alongside me. The distraction of having a new person to talk to was always welcome, and they would often open up about what had made them decide to join me that day. It was a privilege to get so many glimpses into other people's lives.

One of the most surprising things that I heard repeatedly on these runs was that it was the people closest to them – their parents, friends or partner – who were a limitation. We can often be our own worst critics and doubt our ability to do things, especially when we see what everyone else is doing on social media. And hearing it from the people around us can reinforce that lack of self-belief.

There was one guy who ran with me for a few miles who told me about how his girlfriend had dumped him two marathons into the twelve he had set himself that year. She'd complained about his lack of energy at times, and his desire not to do certain things like going out drinking. If another of his friends had backed up what she was saying, he might have given up on his goal.

What he'd really needed to hear from his partner was that what he was doing was unbelievable, that it had value and that he should persist with it and not be deterred when things got hard. Sometimes, when it comes to the people closest to us, particularly our partners, it is a gift to find out soon that they aren't going to be the sort of person who supports us in our goals. It's much better to find out early on, rather than six months or even years down the line, after getting married, having children or starting a business together. Even a negative experience of separating from a partner can teach us a valuable lesson.

The doubts and worries of our loved ones feel like limitations but they can also come from a place of love, care and protectiveness. A girl I met through the gym and started to support in her running, Imogen, told me her friends and family weren't too keen on her running from John O'Groats to Land's End. She had been battling an eating disorder for years and had finally pulled through. But after spending so long worrying about her, those closest to Imogen had found it difficult to stop. They thought she might get hurt running so far. Their concern came from a place of love but to her it felt like they were holding her back. Fortunately, Imogen found the strength to push past that and became the youngest female to run the route she did. Because of that, Nike later flew her out to America to give a panel talk about what she had achieved. I find her story so inspirational – not just because of the battles she fought in the past, but because of how she overcame the doubters and trusted herself.

It makes me wonder how many people in the world right now have been given a gift they will never find out about. They have listened to the doubters and, as a result, not had the opportunity to discover their true potential. Our environment – the people who surround us – has so much influence on whether we pursue our dreams or not. If all you've ever heard are limitations, you will begin to believe them. Your ambition may seem impossible to others, but all that matters is whether you have the faith that you can do it.

Maybe 99 per cent of your environment is currently telling you no. Perhaps what you need to find is a yes.

Lesson 6:
Do Listen to the People You Trust

It was the sixteenth day of the John O'Groats to Land's End challenge, and we had just crossed into Devon. We were seriously behind, as the fatigue had kicked in and there were a few recent days where we hadn't covered our target of 50 miles a day. When we crossed into Devon, we had to push even harder to make up the distance and reach 60 miles in one day.

By late afternoon there were still 8 miles to go, but I couldn't give up or the whole challenge timetable would slip. At times I was hallucinating, vomiting or having full-body convulsions. It was horrendous. I honestly thought it was over, and I wouldn't reach that 60-mile mark.

But I also had Kris King in my team, who was an experienced ultra-athlete himself. Rather than letting me cut it short and rebuild for the next day like I wanted to, he kept on pushing and pushing me. Whenever I reached out to press that metaphorical big red button we all have when we want to stop doing something, he wouldn't let me. He kept pulling my hand back and telling me to go a little further, much to my dismay.

After miles of agony, something extraordinary happened when we hit mile 55. I'd gone through such a level of pain, exhaustion and fatigue that my unconscious mind seemed to take over. A burst of energy came from nowhere, and I went from 3 miles an hour to 15 miles an hour and held that for the final 5 miles. My mind was sharp, and suddenly the route I needed to take along the roads was clear. I zoomed through the lanes, Kris following close behind me on a bicycle. Then we hit the 60-mile mark and Kris called out, telling me to stop. I shook myself out of the trance state I had been in, my emotions decompressed, and I burst into tears. I turned to Kris and asked him what had happened to me and he responded, 'That's what you call flow state, my man.'

I can only describe it as going through a barrier into a place you've never been before. You are completely alert and focused and feel like you can continue with what you're doing forever because you have a superhuman amount of energy within you.

Every time I feel broken now, I reflect on moments like that and how I had more to give. I also know that if I didn't have Kris with me that day – someone who I trusted – I wouldn't have completed that challenge in time. Because he was so experienced in this field from his years as an ultra-runner and owning a successful ultra-events company, he knew that my body was capable of much more.

If I had stopped, I would have wondered for the rest of my life whether I did so because I needed to stop or because my mind had overruled my body. That's the thing about pushing the big red button – it provides momentary relief, but it can get in the way of the satisfaction of going one step further and completing something much bigger than you ever thought you could achieve.

This is another example of how the people around you can impact your life. I trusted Kris, and I was rewarded. Equally, if Kris had told me to stop, I would have. If you ever want to push yourself to the limit, you need to surround yourself with people you trust who know how far you can go. But you also need them there to pull you back when you can't see things as clearly. You can't always make the right decisions for yourself.

Kris had already proven himself earlier on in the challenge, when we had gone from quieter countryside roads to facing a hectic roundabout. It was the first time I had experienced being around a large number of cars in my wheelchair, and fear took over as I felt really vulnerable. Calling the team together, I told them we would break for the day and tackle the roundabout the following morning after some sleep. Kris stepped up and pushed back. He told me that, with the greatest respect, if I was scared today, I would still be scared tomorrow. As the team leader, he wanted us to face this problem head-on and make sure our timetable didn't slip because of it.

When I woke the following day, knowing that I had tackled that tricky roundabout and carried on for a few miles afterwards, I was incredibly grateful to Kris for having pushed me to take that approach. I was also quite proud of myself for listening to him and considering it from his point of view. I could have pulled rank on him, said it was my challenge and I called the shots, but that would have discounted his expertise. It would have reduced him to someone who drove the car behind us when he had so much more to offer. By listening to him, it was me who ultimately benefited.

This is of course a very specific example, but listening to the people you trust is crucial, whatever your purpose in life is. It might be the dance teacher who enters you into a local competition, the colleague who shows you how to use a new bit of software you need for a promotion, or the friend who helps you set up a side hustle. I'm lucky to have people I trust in many areas of my life, and there are other people where if I had listened to their views on my career early on, I wouldn't have done a quarter of the things I've managed to achieve.

The key is that we are listening to people we *trust*. They must have our best interests at heart, and we must be sure that they not only care about our immediate well-being, but also our long-term goals.

A perfect example of this came up early in the 76 Marathons challenge. For Marathon 9 in Bangor in Wales, I had to wear an ankle support because my Achilles tendon was in such a bad way. What I didn't know at the time was that the ankle support shifted my foot, so I was loading my weight onto its side. Soon there was a lot of pain in the base of my foot too. And it didn't end there, because later on in the challenge the calf muscle of my other leg became incredibly painful. There is video footage of Marathon 40 of me turning to the cameraman and telling him that I was in a sticky situation. My right leg didn't want me to put weight on it and was trying to push the weight to the other leg. The weight would go over to my injured left foot, and then it would shift it straight back to the right leg.

I had known I would get injured during this challenge – immediate pain was inevitable, and I had gone into it with full awareness of this – but I didn't want that fact to prevent me from finishing the challenge if I could avoid it. By surrounding myself with people who I trusted, I was able to take a specific approach to my injuries. Before we started, I sat the team down and had a heartfelt discussion where I told them we knew I would get injured, but I didn't want to know the actual diagnosis. Instead, I wanted my physio, Charlie, to know what he was dealing with but only tell me about it at the end of the challenge. All I wanted to know while I was running was how to approach it each day, and how to make the pain bearable. There was one other condition to my request. If at any stage my injuries looked like they would do permanent damage and lifelong harm, then we would have to stop the challenge. We would only continue while the damage was reversible. The team agreed to this, and I put my health in their hands. It wasn't until the end that I found out the extent of my injuries.

My view of success isn't about money or beating other people. It's about surrounding myself with the best people who can help me be the best version of myself. On this occasion, my trusted team showed me how passionate they were about my goals and would often put me first, before themselves. They'd drop everything and travel to meet me if they thought I needed the support, whether mental or physical. This is the difference between the doubters and the people you trust who care about you and want the best for you. Having my team in my corner kept me going, and in the end, this world record was for them. Even though I was the person awarded it, every one of them was part of it too. Without each individual who was part of that experience, I wouldn't have achieved my goal. It is as much their record as it is mine, and I got there by listening to them.

Lesson 7: A Diagnosis Can be a Blessing or a Curse

I watched as my trusted physiotherapist, Charlie, strapped up my leg. He had travelled down to Chichester to treat me and then complete his first marathon by my side. My other physical therapist, Sharon, had also travelled across the country a few times during the course of the 76 Marathons so far. She had even flown up to Scotland on short notice when the pain in my foot started getting really bad. Between them both, they had kept me patched up. I had told them and the rest of the team not to let me know about the diagnosis for my foot and calf unless the damage was irreversible, and they had kept to their word. So, I pulled on my trainers, opened the door to the camper van, and set off on my sixty-seventh marathon, this time with Charlie running alongside me.

I didn't want to know what I had done to myself because I was fully aware of the power those diagnoses would have on my mental state. I knew the truth would weigh on my mind and make it harder to push through the pain. It wasn't until I completed all 76 marathons that the team would sit me down and explain that, since Marathon 9, I had been running on a stress fracture in my foot, and since Marathon 40, I had been running with a torn calf muscle in my other leg. It sounds crazy to think that now, but I finished without causing any long-term damage to my body, so I made the right decision to remain oblivious of the exact details.

Through trusting my team, I could wake up each morning and accept the pain because I knew it was temporary and I would recover after the challenge. It would have been a very different outcome if I'd been told on Marathon 9 that I had a stress fracture. With every step I took, every time my foot connected with the ground, I would have wondered if I was damaging it more. It would have been this thought that played on my mind for the rest of each day.

The mind is a powerful thing; it interprets reality and plays it back to us, and can even fabricate it in the process. This is why it can be a blessing not to know the full truth, because when our brain isn't aware of something it can be our champion and keep pushing us forward. Whereas when it is alerted to something potentially detrimental, it can easily become fixated on it in an effort to protect us. For me, in my unique situation, deciding not to be told the whole truth was the best choice to make, and it kept me going. In other cases, the right approach will be different.

It is human nature to want to know the truth and diagnose ourselves whenever we notice something that isn't quite right. Particularly when it comes to mental health, it can be such a blessing to get that validation, but it can also be a curse.

A psychologist once told me that they would be cautious about diagnosing someone with a mental health condition because of the two very different approaches patients can take. Some people view having a name for a set of symptoms as life-changing in the most freeing way. They have usually gone through a significant period knowing that something isn't quite right but unaware of what it is, what it means or how to make the best of it. To be given a diagnosis lifts a weight from their shoulders. But for others, the minute they are diagnosed and labelled with something, it can feel overwhelming, as though they are defined by that condition. This isn't to say that they don't have the strength to deal with it. But they might not be given any understanding of what their diagnosis really means, or they might not have a supportive environment to empower them to embrace it and make the most of it. They can become a victim of their diagnosis.

For a long time, I have suspected I might have ADHD. I have all the signs of it, and unlike when I was determined to push through the pain of my injuries during the 76 Marathons without a diagnosis, I do want to find out. What has stopped me – which might be another sign of ADHD – is that I am struggling to get around to organizing the process of being properly tested – which, according to a shocking recent report, can take up to ten years. My desire for a diagnosis is my decision and my chosen approach. Others might want to take a different route, and may feel they don't need or want an official diagnosis. It is about knowing yourself and anticipating your own reaction.

Choosing whether to pursue a diagnosis for certain conditions is just one of the many choices we make that can positively or negatively affect our mindset, something we'll cover in the next chapter.

Lesson 8: Your Choices Will Impact Your Situation or Mindset

A friend of mine had messaged to ask if we could chat about the progress he had been making in the gym. When we finally spoke, he told me he was feeling pretty demoralized as he wasn't seeing the results he had anticipated. This was despite having a personalized plan and going to the gym religiously four days a week for a few months. He'd reached a plateau and couldn't understand why he wasn't making further progress.

With dedication like that, it didn't make much sense to me either, so I asked him what he was doing outside of the gym. He told me about his diet and it was clear he wasn't eating very healthily and was drinking regularly. There was no judgement from me on this. I understand the pressure that people are under and how easy it is to reach for something that seems to instantly lighten it, but that is a short-term solution that might cause more damage in the long term, so it's worth thinking about the underlying motivation for reaching out for such things in the first place.

Just having that chat made my friend think more about his approach. He realized that he had a decision to make. He could either carry on as he was, or decide to increase the nutritional content of the food he was eating and cut down on his drinking. It was his choice, and what he decided would control the outcome. He made up his mind that he wasn't finished reaching his exercise goal and wanted to make further changes to see where they would take him.

It might be because I've been very aware of my mental health for most of my life (which I'll talk more about later), but at a young age I realized that every choice I make will either positively or negatively affect my situation or mindset – from the big things like my career and productivity, right down to the small things like my daily habits. With things like food and alcohol, I started to see the common patterns and how choosing to indulge when I was feeling low could make me feel good in the moment, but would later negatively affect how I felt, looked or performed, and so ultimately bring me down further. I began to see the clear link between action and outcome, which helped me to choose whether to do something or say no.

If I want to have a body that is energetic and able to do what I ask of it, I have to feed it the right food regularly. If I want to make the most of my day, I probably won't drink alcohol the night before. If I want to keep my anxiety under control, I need quality sleep most nights and also to take into account my drinking and food intake. With nearly every decision I face, I try to weigh up the instant gratification versus the longer-term impact.

This has allowed me to recognize when I take one

approach a bit too far. Sometimes I have trained too hard and forgotten it's about enjoying the process, so I've pulled it back. After completing a challenge, I eat what I want for a few weeks as a nice transition, but that eventually comes to a natural end because I know that my body needs more nutritious food.

Life is about balance and finding a bit of joy alongside your accomplishments. As we'll cover in the next chapter, it doesn't mean you have to go all in one way or the other. It's about weighing up the potential outcomes and making the right choice for you at that time. Wanting to be more healthy, for example, doesn't mean that you can't enjoy a night out with your friends or have fun. Those evenings out can be a wonderful thing – maybe even one of those legendary nights you're still talking about five years later. It's not about having a perfect diet either. It's about putting the power back in your own hands and making more conscious decisions, rather than being ruled by your emotions or by bad habits. Go on that night out or have that takeaway after a long draining week at work. Absorb every bit of joy from it, and allow it to lift you up so that you feel content and fulfilled, and ready to take on the next day or week and make great choices for yourself. When you act from a place of control rather than desperation, you can make better choices.

You are in control of your future by controlling your here and now, so make every decision count.

Lesson 9: Balance is the Key to Longevity

In the two months following the 76 Marathons, I only ran a couple of times. That wasn't because I was sick of running and couldn't face it anymore. It was because, after the first couple of runs, there was no sign of improvement with the stress fracture in my foot, so I was advised by my team not to continue running while it healed. I'd been told that it wasn't a permanent injury, but it could still get progressively worse if I didn't rest enough.

At this point, I had to make a tough decision to preserve my own longevity. It was a case of prioritizing the recovery process over my short-term desperation to get the best results. Three years before, I'd hated running, but over time I fell in love with it and found not being able to run incredibly frustrating. Having pushed through so many mental barriers and achieved things that I'd never thought possible, it was hard to finally be told that I had to stop. That was difficult to come to terms with, but I realized there was nothing to be gained from pushing, and a lot to be lost. I knew that if I wanted to be able to run in the long term, I had to listen to my body and the experts. So, my focus shifted to strength and conditioning work in the gym until I was given the all-clear. I wanted to ensure that I'd taken all precautions, so I could continue with a sport that I loved.

When we discover what we can achieve, it can be tempting to push ourselves and take it too far. We can get impatient and cut corners in order to move on to the next goal, medal, competition, step or stage. Sometimes we treat this activity or skill that we are so passionate about as a way of stimulating and distracting our minds to block out everything else that is going on. It becomes a new fixation to numb us to a previous one (that's perhaps another aspect of my ADHD brain, but hopefully you can relate). Depending on what we are trying to achieve, the repercussions can be far-ranging, and our body, relationships, social life, or finances can take the hit.

Things can quickly spiral when we first become passionate about something, and it can be easy to confuse a determined mindset with a balanced one. I have seen this a lot in the fitness space and have even fallen into this way of thinking a couple of times myself. People start a fitness regime, and within a few weeks they've completely cut out bread and villainized white rice. It's a cycle of cut, bulk and shred, which is so easy to get pulled into because social media is filled with athletes and fitness influencers explaining how they achieved their body shape. They post about every aspect of their day because they need content, and people viewing that content can become fixated. Those athletes and influencers don't necessarily expect those watching to live the same way, but viewers often think that's what they're supposed to do. The problem is that their lifestyle is not everybody's lifestyle, and some of us are led to try to achieve something that's not achievable for us. We don't take into account the differences in ability, environment and responsibilities. So when we try to reproduce these individuals' behaviour patterns, the synergy is not there, and it can negatively affect how we view our own progress.

Unfortunately, we can't always match what others do. If you're a mother or father and you've heard that you should be up at 5 a.m. to train, but your child has kept you up all night, that is simply not realistic. If you're religiously trying to follow that structure, it will negatively impact you and potentially your relationships. You could easily lose confidence and then blame yourself because you cannot fulfil someone else's aspirations.

I can, hand on heart, say that I would have ended the 76 Marathons challenge if I'd incurred an injury that would have caused irreversible damage to my body. It would have crushed me, but I still would have pulled out. It would have been the end of the challenge even if a few rest days would have been enough for my recovery, because the marathons had to be consecutive. The goal at the time was running a marathon in every UK city in 76 days, and I had to push myself mentally and physically to get there, but my long-term goal is to keep on doing challenges to raise money and awareness for charities. I can only do that by sometimes taking my foot off the gas and prioritizing my longevity. It's hard to always get this balance right, but I've learned that it is the key to a long, fulfilling life.

Lesson 10: Listen to the Warning Signals

I watched the video we had created for an Instagram reel again and decided we couldn't use it. In every single shot, I was either mumbling, grimacing or staring blankly at the camera. Not exactly riveting viewing. The footage was of Marathon 63, in Winchester, and I'd had no energy left, so instead of the video I chose some photos for the post that showed just how drained I was. We had been on the road for almost ten weeks, and I had woken up that morning and had sincerely not wanted to run. It felt like there was nothing else to give.

I felt guilty that people were showing up to run with us each day and I was struggling to have my usual chats with them. Normally, I looked forward to meeting and connecting with new people, but I was finding it difficult to have the simplest conversations, even with my team. My cognitive functions had begun to be affected, and my speech was slurred. For everyone who came to run with me, I wanted to ensure that it was a real experience for them, but I was unable to fulfil that aim consistently. I'd felt buried inside myself that day and wasn't able to emerge. Something had to change.

My mind and body were telling me something wasn't right, and I had to take some time to myself to reset. So,

I got out my phone and found a local gym to visit. When I tell people that I sometimes go to the gym after running a marathon, they often look at me with concern. But the gym is a place of peace for me that always helps my mental health, and I needed somewhere relaxing if I wanted to reset. I lifted some weights and felt my mindset adjust.

That short time away from things gave me a chance to recover. The following day was Milton Keynes, where my energy levels soared, and I ran my fastest marathon time since starting the challenge. The phoenix within had risen again! And because I had approached it with a completely different mindset to the previous day, I got so much more out of it. It was rocket fuel. Winchester had been the warning from my body and mind, and in Milton Keynes was the polar opposite.

I always try to listen to my body and mind when they tell me something isn't right. If I'm bloated, it's for a reason. If I'm tired, it's for a reason. I try to ask myself why I feel like this and give an honest answer. It's only when we understand a situation that we have a chance to improve it. It's then up to us whether we are kind enough to ourselves to do anything about it.

Like anyone who has been diagnosed with depression and anxiety, I'm always alert to whether they will affect me. When I start to notice the warning signs, I make some quick adjustments, so they can't pull me down. Resetting usually involves something small that will help my mood. It could be a gym visit, eating food with friends, or just FaceTiming them if we can't meet up. It doesn't have to be anything big or extravagant.

Occasionally, though, I need more help with resetting my mind, in which case I visit a woman who has always managed to help me in those moments . . .

Lesson 11: Anxiety is Normal When Challenging Yourself

Once again, I found myself sitting in the therapy room of one of the most soothing women I know – exactly what a mental health specialist should be. I knew that if I had any issue in the world, I could take it to her, and by the time I left her office, my day would be lit up again. A medical doctor who combines therapy and coaching, her approach is very holistic. The world would be a very different place if everyone had someone like her in their lives.

It was 10 a.m., and I was trying to explain to her through a foggy mind that I thought I was depressed again. All the signs were there and I began ticking them off on my fingers: tiredness, anxious thoughts, insomnia, not wanting to get up in the morning, low mood, and a lack of interest in things. The list went on. She asked what was going on in my life beyond how I was feeling, and carefully listened as I told her about a situation where I thought I was being portrayed in an unjust way in an environment I found to be incredibly toxic. Before she'd even said anything, I could feel that just having someone to talk to about it was helping – I didn't feel so weighed down. When I had finished, she asked, 'How would you feel if I instantly took this issue away from you?' I immediately responded that I would feel a hell of a lot better. She went on to ask, 'Would you still feel all these things you've described?' I thought about it for a moment before responding that I didn't believe I would. 'Then you're not depressed,' she said carefully. 'You're situationally unhappy. Which means that it's about your environment rather than what's happening internally.'

This was a revolutionary moment for me. I have been diagnosed with depression in the past, and naturally, like anyone who has had an illness, I have always feared it coming back again. To hear that what I was going through at that time was not depression, but instead the impact of my environment, was transformative.

The same goes for my anxiety. Sometimes I'm anxious because I am an anxious person and it can build up out of nowhere and in relation to nothing, but sometimes it is because of the situation I'm in. It doesn't mean I am going through a full-blown period of anxiety where I worry about anything and everything. Whenever I am going through a tough time now, I always think about how I would feel if a particular issue was resolved. Thankfully, I have always found that when I imagine that scenario, I feel much better, and my anxiety can be managed.

I quickly learned that the same applied to the challenges I set for myself. Before a challenge, I would find myself sleeping less and sometimes worrying into the night. For a time, I thought maybe my mental health conditions were returning, but then I realized that feeling more stressed and anxious is normal while I am preparing for them. The logistics are often huge and come with many variables. These challenges require me to be intently focused on the future and, for me, that often causes anxious thoughts.

It's natural to have nerves when we're about to do something we've never attempted before, but it is within our power to control how we respond to those nerves, and sometimes we have to tailor our approach to make the challenge feel more doable. My sister's experience with running is the perfect example of this. She recently started running and set herself the goal of running 10 kilometres. She completed all of her training, but when it came to running the full distance, she was anxious about it, and it had built up into a huge hurdle in her mind. When we spoke about this, I told her that she was missing out on the joy of running. Something that was supposed to be such a beneficial experience had become something that was having a negative impact. We agreed that rather than running the 10 kilometres on a treadmill, which she thought she should do, she would do it in an environment that made her happy. She chose a beautiful lake we had run around during the Norwich day of the 76 Marathons. A few days later, she called me to announce that she had done it. By tailoring her environment and the situation to suit her, she had overcome her anxiety surrounding achieving her goal and turned it into enjoyment.

The magical thing is that these types of worries often

disappear when you hit the start line. All that built-up anticipation suddenly has a release, and you are intently focused on what you are doing and the joy that comes with it. When I was doing the 76 Marathons, for two and a half months I didn't have any anxiety. At times I was exhausted, injured, in a lot of pain or withdrawn, but never anxious. I was in the moment, focusing on the here and now, doing something I loved; and there was a fixed structure to every day. There were no complications. I would wake up, I would eat my breakfast, I would run, I would recover, and then we'd go again the next day. It was a million miles away from everyday life, which has become so complicated. All those day-to-day responsibilities were eradicated during that challenge, and my mind was free to focus on just putting one foot in front of the other. The energy of the people around me also helped. We were doing such a positive thing together; we had a shared purpose and other positive people were drawn to the challenge – it was the law of attraction.

Unfortunately, that high couldn't last, and within an hour of returning to London for the last two marathons, I began biting the skin around my nails, which I hadn't done for two and a half months. My body tensed up, and my mind was darting from one thing to the next. The change was instantaneous. Even though I was still focused on finishing the challenge, the intensity of the environment was affecting my mental state.

I knew in that moment that London was a trigger for my anxiety. This could have been upsetting, but I soon realized that knowing that fact gave me the power to control it. Strangely, it actually makes me feel better that I can reduce my struggles with anxiety if I take myself out of that city environment. It makes it feel less permanent and provides a temporary solution. It might not be one I can use all the time at the moment because London is where my life is, but I'm not going to be like this forever. One day in the future I will probably return to the countryside. In the meantime, I can leave a few times a month and find a place of peace, and my anxiety will improve.

Just like the anxiety and worry that can build up when you face challenges in life or do something outside of your comfort zone, there will be outside factors that can impact your mental health. But when you know what they are, and know they aren't inherent in you, they won't have so much power.

Lesson 12: Don't be Too Proud to Reach Out for Help

As somebody who has struggled with their mental health from a young age, I know how hard it can be to seek help. As I talked about earlier, I decided to run 76 marathons in 76 days around the 76 cities in the UK where the Samaritans have offices. So many people still struggle to accept when they need help, so my mission was to empower them to seek that help.

I knew all those marathons would be extremely challenging and push me to my limits. I become vulnerable when I reach my limits, as we all do, and I wanted men in particular to know that it's okay to be vulnerable and to feel overwhelmed sometimes. It's just part of being human. What's more damaging is if we always try to pretend that everything is fine or that we aren't feeling anything. That just isn't sustainable in the long run, and won't lead to a fulfilling life full of thriving relationships.

This is something I learned much earlier than many others, and although it came out of a difficult time, I am grateful for that early life lesson. I first had therapy at around twelve or thirteen years old, when my parents were getting divorced and I was unable to understand my emotions. I didn't know whether what I was feeling was anxiety, anger or fear. I had tried everything in my power to make sure that my parents were happy, but I knew it wasn't enough. My world was about to change forever, and I had no real idea what that new world would be like.

I was old enough to understand the possible implications of their separation on me and my family but too young to be able to process it properly or feel like I had any control over my situation. There was no way out for me, and I couldn't just pack up and go away for a few days as I might do now. I was stuck right there, in the eye of the storm. The most confusing thing was that they announced they were going to get a divorce, and then nothing happened. On the surface, it was as if that conversation had never occurred, and the sense of responsibility I felt to keep my parents happy increased. Inside I felt scared, and my home didn't feel like a stable place.

Eventually, they did proceed with the divorce and my dad moved to Norfolk while I stayed in Lincolnshire with my mum and sister. I then moved to Norfolk to live with my dad as I didn't want him to be alone, and it took me an hour and a half to get to school each way. Soon after that, my behaviour both at school and towards my parents began to worsen. I started getting into trouble and was suspended. I was lucky to have parents who loved me and were aware of how their decision had impacted me, and I had a very understanding head-teacher, Mr Clifford, so I think between them it was decided that I needed to see a therapist.

I wish I could tell you that my first experience of therapy was a great success and that, after a few sessions, I skipped out of there, newly balanced and adjusted. But that was not the case. The thing about therapy that isn't talked about enough is that it's a partnership, and if the synergy and trust aren't there, it won't work. It doesn't matter how professional or experienced a therapist is, it's not human nature to open up to someone we don't feel comfortable around. What I remember about those first few sessions is just being really pissed off at the world. I was furious and resentful about everything, including being expected to talk about my feelings. It was clear it wasn't going to work out so, before long, that first therapist was replaced by an amazing one who I instantly clicked with. Just being in the same room as her calmed me down, and this allowed me to start thinking less about how annoyed I was with everything and everyone else, and focus more on what was happening to me. I instinctively knew I could trust her, and that allowed me to begin to open up. I learned that part of what I was feeling was shame that I was the first kid I knew who this had happened to, and that we had lost the family's friendship group and our family home. It felt as though we were tainted. My therapist was the first person to let me know that what I was feeling was normal.

Looking back on it, I might have been suppressing quite a bit of what I was feeling, but I was young and wanted to appear like I was okay. I've had therapy at different stages of my life, and I still go back to this same therapist. I've now reached a point where I can be completely truthful about what I'm feeling with her, as I know from experience that this is the only way to get the work done.

I'm lucky to have experienced the benefits of therapy from a young age, but I know it's not easy to take that step later in life. I could write a whole book on the reasons why it's so great, but to keep it short, I'm just going to focus on two.

First, it makes you feel settled and content, which is a truckload better than chasing 'happiness'. From going to therapy I've learned that happiness is a subjective feeling without an end point, whereas feeling content and settled in yourself is so much more achievable and comforting. Without that grounding you can feel like you are constantly chasing something or turning to potentially damaging behaviours to block out or dull what you're feeling. Both of these impulses can be pretty destructive if left unchecked.

The second is that it teaches you how to express yourself, which is such a fundamental and life-changing skill – so much so that it should be taught in schools. If you can express yourself and convey what you are feeling or what you need, it will have a positive impact that ripples out to all your relationships. How many situations flare up at home, with friends or at work because you are unable to communicate properly and someone has misinterpreted what you were trying to say? It happens all the time, and the consequences can be life-changing if we don't have the skills to repair the situation. But when we express ourselves properly, we can feel heard, understood and closer to the people around us. And perhaps that's all we ever really need – to be closer to people. To be understood.

Some people still think that going to therapy means you are weak. That if you seek help, you are closer to breaking than you should be, that you are on a downward spiral and are somehow not quite whole. You might have sat next to one of the people who believe this in the pub recently and had a pint with them, or you might be in a relationship with one. You might even have held this belief yourself or still do.

I know there might not be much I can say to change those people's opinions, but it's my belief that by seeking help, not only will you become a better version of yourself, but you will get more out of your relationships and more people will be drawn to you. All you need is one productive relationship with a therapist to enable all those other potential positive relationships to happen. I really believe that seeking professional help doesn't make us weak. It's quite the opposite – it makes us strong.

Lesson 13: There is No Such Thing as Failure, Only a Lesson to be Learned

Around a year ago, my finger hovered over the 'post' button as I imagined all the possible outcomes of making that one tiny movement and releasing a message to the world. It was a photo of me where I didn't think I looked that great. My muscle loss over the past few months was clear to see, and my chest and back were covered in psoriasis from the stress I'd been under. But the photo wasn't what bothered me so much, although I wasn't happy with what I saw in the mirror each day. What made me hesitate were the words that accompanied the photo. For the first time in years, I was about to tell the world I couldn't do something I had set out to achieve. I knew in some people's eyes, they would view it as a failure.

In the running community, there is a golden achievement for middle-distance runners – a kind of solo expedition up Everest which many aim for and only a few achieve. It is the four-minute mile. Sir Roger Bannister was the first person to achieve it, in 1954, at the age of twenty-five. Before then, it was always thought impossible for anyone to run a mile in under four minutes. Like many things in life, once Roger proved it could be done, it opened up mental blocks for so many other runners, and a couple of months later, two others managed it. Over the next seventy years, around 1,800 other runners joined them, and I had decided I wanted to be one of them.

Looking back, I now realize that my Why at the time was for all the wrong reasons. Normally I set myself challenges because I love running and want to help people. This one started out because I was inspired by Roger Bannister and those who followed in his footsteps, but it quickly became wrapped up in my ego. Some people on social media, rather than supporting me, would tell me I couldn't do it. That cut deep but also fired up my ego, and it became more about proving them wrong than enjoying the process. So I trained hard and kept on pushing myself. Eventually, I trained myself into an injury, and that's where the issue I would later face with my Achilles tendon came from. I would train, re-injure myself, rest, train, re-injure myself. We kept pushing back the date of my four-minute-mile attempt, and my mental health progressively got worse. I wasn't sleeping properly, I was biting my nails and having anxious thoughts. I lost my motivation and stopped training.

On the day I published that post, I knew something had to change and I had to be honest about my situation. A few weeks before, I had admitted to myself that I couldn't run a four-minute mile with my injuries, and removing that pressure should have made me feel lighter, but my confidence took a knock. I had gotten the process fundamentally wrong, and both my mind and my body were paying the price. I knew I had two choices. I could either live in the past in my perceived failure or look at what could be next.

I tried not to treat it as a failure, even though part of my mind sometimes viewed it that way. Instead, I looked at what I could learn from it – what were the lessons I could take away? I ditched the mentality that I would only train to improve my running and started broadening out the exercises I was doing. Gradually my mindset shifted away from a laser focus on training and eating to enhance my running performance. This meant that when I went into the 76 Marathons, it was with a completely different mindset.

I believe that instead of there being successes and failures, there are successes and lessons. The lesson from my four-minute-mile training was that I had taken the joy out of my Why. I had never wanted to run to try to beat a time before, as it affects my mental health. Yet, somehow, I had thrown myself into training for the lowest time imaginable.

Not completing something doesn't mean it's the end of your journey – it just leads to another path if you decide to look for it. It was partly because of that experience – that 'failure' – that I felt reinvigorated and went back to training to run 76 marathons in 76 days for the first time in two years. That experience of *not* achieving the thing I had set out to taught me so much more than if I had achieved it. It changed everything for me, and I decided I was going to approach the 76 Marathons in a completely different way. Now I try not to be disheartened by the setbacks in life, because they are usually there to steer you in a better direction. There's no such thing as failure, only lessons to be learned.

Lesson 14: Recovery is as Important as Performance

When my team first explained the plan they had created to get me through daily marathons for two and a half months, it was not what I'd expected. It blew my mind that running wouldn't be the major priority when we were preparing for the greatest challenge of my life. But I trusted my team of experts, and it was actually quite touching that their main focus for this endeavour was to keep me injury-free. After the constant injuries that had dogged me throughout my four-minute-mile training, I knew my current approach wasn't working. We needed to bring in more balance, as running would improve my fitness but also potentially worsen any injury I had previously sustained.

The problems I had faced in the previous challenge largely came from overtraining – but, equally, I wasn't looking after my body. Right from the beginning, I had taken a 110 per cent approach to these challenges. In a way, it was self-destructive – but in what I thought was a really constructive way. When I was struggling with my mental health, rather than turn to classic distractions like junk food, TV, alcohol or drugs, I had thrown myself into my challenges. Looking back now, I can see that my approach to them began as a type of self-harm.

If I was going to hurt myself, I had decided, I wanted to do it in a way that made me feel good about what I was doing. It wasn't as if I wanted to find something socially acceptable to mask what I was trying to do to myself. It was more that I wanted to throw myself into something where I could let my frustrations out. But that wasn't healthy. And it also wasn't constructive, because it had a short life, and my body had started paying the price for it.

I've seen a similar approach in other people who exercise a lot. They finish up a challenge or achieve a goal they set themselves, and immediately throw themselves into the next one without pausing for a moment to take care of themselves. Rather than making mobility, nutrition and sleep their priority, they plough on with training and then question why it takes them so long to recover and be ready for the next mission. It took me years to accept that if I prioritized these key things rather than a new training routine, my recovery progress would actually speed up.

So, we had a new plan and a new approach, in which my recovery was as important as my performance. With age and experience now on my side, I embraced this transition rather than throwing myself into preparing for my challenge as a way of escaping anything else happening in my life. For the first time, I would be focusing more on strength and conditioning in the gym. I had done strength and conditioning work before, but nothing to this level. The game changer was that we were trying to build up my body in a different way, to prepare it to withstand the prolonged impact that I was going to sustain for the 76 days. I would also be spending around five hours a week with physios, osteopaths and sports therapists. It was this alternative approach that would ultimately get me through my longest challenge.

I'm really proud that I made that change, because I see 'destructive in the name of constructive' behaviour in a lot of people. So many of us adopt it because we think it's what we should be doing. We graft, we give 100 per cent, we burn the candle at both ends and work long days because we're told that is what success looks like. If, during this time, we feel tired, we might even begin to wonder if we're lazy. I read a quote recently that summed up this idea perfectly: 'Rather than thinking that I'm lazy, perhaps I should ask myself why I'm so tired.'

Maybe whatever you are challenging yourself with or prioritizing doesn't involve much exercise. But you will still need recovery time if it takes up a lot of your day; it's just that your recovery might look different. It might be that what you are doing, such as a new job or study-ing, means you have to sit down for long amounts of time, in which case your recovery might be doing some gentle exercise such as going for a walk. Or if you're a parent, you might need some quiet time to yourself, or a few hours each week to do other things in your life – you can't be a fun playful parent all the time.

Recovery looks different depending on what we spend most of our time doing, but it's always about loving our body and being thankful for what it does for us. My challenges have taught me to be grateful for my body and that it is able to do what I ask of it, even though it would probably prefer something a bit more relaxing, with the odd rest day.

It's so easy to take our bodies for granted and just expect them to perform for us because they are so powerful and resilient. But if you don't look after your body, one day it will break. Therefore, its recovery is as important as its performance.

Lesson 15: Live with Gratitude

I reached a point in my early twenties where I was unbelievably lost and I spiralled to the lowest I have ever felt. As a warning, there are references to self-harm in this chapter, so please feel free to skip it if you think that could negatively affect you.

I had always wanted a career as a professional rugby player, and fought hard to join a team in Northern Ireland, where my dad's family are from. I had originally been on a team in London but hadn't been supported by the coach there, and I'd felt frustrated by the politics which meant that players who weren't as good as me were being picked before me. Because I'm very confident, it was perceived as arrogance by the coach, and he thought he had to beat it out of me. So, I wanted to find a new team and get a fresh start. When I joined my team in Northern Ireland, it seemed like my dreams were finally coming true. Only, it didn't go the way I'd expected. My debut game was great and I scored an amazing try, so I didn't understand the coach's reasoning when he didn't pick me for the first team for the next game. Because of this, my anxiety began crippling my performance on the pitch. It got to the stage where I was so nervous and overwhelmed that I kept dropping the ball. Can you imagine it? I was a professional rugby player who struggled to catch the ball. I started getting moved down the teams until I was on the third team, and after two years my contract wasn't renewed and I knew I wouldn't get another one.

When my rugby career ended, I unknowingly fell into a deep depression. Like many people who have spent their younger years trying to be a professional sportsperson, there was no plan B. I had been completely focused on plan A, and it hadn't worked out. I had achieved what I had set out to do by being picked up by a team, but my dream had been cut short because of my mental health. Once I lost my place on the team, I didn't know what to do with myself. I felt like my life was over at twenty-two.

This was the absolute lowest point of my life. I was living with my mum because my relationship with my dad was so difficult at the time. I wouldn't go to bed until four or five in the morning, and then I would sleep until three or four in the afternoon.

Although my relationship with him was challenging during this time, my dad owned a successful building company and, to try to get me out of this rut, he offered me a job as a labourer. He was a self-made man, and having grown up in absolute poverty he believed in hard work and people proving themselves. He would never have offered me a management role – I didn't deserve it, and there were far more experienced people than me who did. And I'm so thankful that he instilled in me this core value of proving your worth.

So, I hauled bricks across building sites all day to prove my worth to the other labourers and builders. I was grateful for the job because it gave me a reason to get up in the morning and brought a small amount of structure into my life when I really needed it. My dad had always been there at my lowest points in life to lift me up.

At that time, despite having been to therapy in my early teens, I still didn't really know how to process my emotions, and losing my rugby career made it feel like the bottom had fallen out of my world, so I expressed myself through aggression. I would get into fights when I went out and smash things up when I was at home. It's not a reaction I'm particularly proud of, but looking back it was clearly an outward expression of the pain I felt inside.

There was one day when I hit rock bottom and destroyed my bedroom. I'd had an argument with my dad and didn't know how to channel my anger and frustration, so I blew up and upended everything I could, smashing pictures and a mirror. Stopping for a moment, I looked at the chaos around me that I had created and was hit by a wave of indescribable guilt and despair. I picked up a shard of glass and put it to my wrist – I still have the puncture scar now – but paused before going any further.

I don't know why I paused, but it triggered something in me that ultimately saved my life. I knew I couldn't continue down this path of outward and inward destruction. That small pause gave me a moment of clarity, and I was able to pull myself back from the dark place I was in and see another way forward. From that day, a new journey began. It felt like I had been given a second chance, and I began to live with gratitude for what I had. My scar is a reminder of how close I came to ending my life, and how, if I had done so, I would have missed out on all the incredible things that have happened to me since then. It's a reminder to be grateful for every day that I get to spend with my daughter, my family and my friends.

I used to hate that I couldn't control the things that happened around me – I still can't – but on that day, I realized that I could control how I responded to them. Gratitude became a firm part of my belief system. Instead of thinking about what I didn't have, I began to focus on what I did have and the bonuses that came with it. It is so hard to see the bubbles that we've been raised in for what they are. We focus on the negatives, cannot accept the positives, and struggle to put our lives into context and gain perspective. But when we stop and think about all the things we *do* have, it can completely shift our mindset. I have so much gratitude for everything in my life now, especially when I look at where I was mentally and emotionally in my early twenties compared to now.

Living with gratitude has got me through all the tough times that followed that dark time in my life. It hasn't prevented bad things from happening, but it does give me a way of dealing with them. It allows me to focus on what is important, and for people with anxious personalities, this can bring immeasurable relief. It's not a case of dismissing how you feel about something – you have to acknowledge it, or it will be buried and come out at another time – but about searching for the positives.

All my adult life, my greatest fear was following in my parents' footsteps and bringing my child up in a broken home. When my greatest fear was realized and I separated from my daughter's mother, I had a choice to make. I could go through life bitter that my worst fear had come true, feel angry at everything and everyone around me and resentful that I wasn't able to give her the home life I thought she deserved. Or I could work hard to raise her well in different circumstances.

I decided to go with the second option, and now my greatest fear has become my greatest happiness. I look at my daughter and she is the most beautiful little thing with the purest heart, and she approaches everything with such joy. I am so grateful for the life I now have with her in it, and that even though the circumstances aren't as I had imagined, she hasn't been affected by them.

I live each day wanting to know that I have maximized the gifts given to me by using the entirety of my body and mind. If something, God forbid, did happen to me tomorrow, I know that I have made the most of what I was given and done enough in my life to be the role model that my daughter needs from her dad. I hope

I have passed on this sense of gratitude so that she can lead a fulfilling and purposeful life.

There is another element to gratitude, which is so important that it needs its own chapter. It is all about using the past for motivation and to help put the present in perspective . . .

Lesson 16: Memories are Motivation

In 2021, I had just finished a world-first of running a marathon in each of the four countries in the UK within twenty-four hours without any rest or sleep between them. The training for this had been tough, and I knew I needed a break and a chance to reset. I had a stress fracture in my ankle and it had swollen up. It was so bad that I needed my mum to help me undress and get into bed. At one point she had to take me to A&E because I was in so much pain, and I had to use a wheelchair and crutches for a while.

The irony is that during the following year, which I had set aside to recover, I managed to get looped into something which turned out to be the absolute opposite of a rest. I had agreed to help a company who had organized my last challenge by supporting another of their events, in Sri Lanka. I went into it completely unprepared, as I thought I'd just be running an ultra-marathon with a team in Sri Lanka – a nice way to test my fitness and meet some other ultra-runners. There wasn't a competition element to it, so I didn't do a lot of training to prepare. It turned out to be a mixture of one of the most life-affirming and merciless experiences I've ever had.

When I landed in Colombo a couple of days before we were due to start, I stepped out of the air-conditioned airport and realized within seconds that the heat was unbearable. It was thirty-nine degrees and 100 per cent humidity, with no breeze. Even just standing outside in the shade, the sweat was pouring down me – and we would have to run an ultra-marathon in this: 250 kilometres in five days, which meant running between 30 and 60 kilometres per day. I soon realized there was no way of acclimatizing to the heat. I'd made a promise to this company so I'd just have to throw myself into the challenge and see what happened.

On the first day, at 6 a.m., we began our slow jog through the rough terrain that was our route through the Sri Lankan countryside. I don't think any of us was prepared for the toll the heat and humidity would have on our bodies. Within only a few minutes, my heart rate shot up to 170 and remained high for the next six hours until we completed the first leg. My body was working overtime just to keep me moving.

By the end of that first day, I was completely drained, but I didn't get any sleep that night because I was sharing a tent with five other people in unbearable heat, and two of them were snorers. I had managed to get through the day by relying on the resilience I had developed in previous races, but then, on top of physical exhaustion and sleep deprivation, began the daily battle with dehydration. There were water stations in the jungles we were running through, but myself and the other runners who had signed up for the ultra-marathon needed it constantly and we would frequently run out. We also needed electrolytes to replenish the salts we sweated out. This was a juggling act, because if you drank too much salt it would have a detrimental effect. On the first day, one of the runners had nearly died from heat exhaustion. She'd been rushed to hospital and saved with an IV drip. Every few hours, another runner would have to drop out because of the heat, and our group continued to grow smaller. The combination of sleep deprivation, humidity, dehydration, heat and physical exhaustion was just brutal.

When I limped into camp at the end of the third day of running, it was raining heavily, and I went off to find something to eat before dinnertime. The rain was only increasing, and after a few hours there was a flash flood that put our campsite in danger. The organizers arranged with a Buddhist temple that they would give us shelter overnight, and we were driven up into the hills. The temple looked like a concrete car park, complete with concrete floor, pillars and ceiling. It was 10 p.m. when one of the monks kindly showed us where we could sleep. We all lay down in one large concrete room, and it felt like I was the only one who didn't get a minute of sleep.

That night was the biggest test of my mental resilience. I knew I had to run again in a few hours but was more exhausted than I think I had ever been. I hadn't slept properly for days, I hadn't eaten dinner as our camp had been washed away, and I was lying on a concrete floor with around sixty other people. It was one of those moments where I thought there was literally nothing else that could be thrown at me. The next day was our penultimate run, and the longest one yet. I knew I had a choice: I could let it break me, or I could get up in the morning and put one foot in front of the other. I decided I would make sure I was ready to run again.

I woke up from my shallow sleep the next morning to a mixture of panic and relief amongst the crew and runners, as the route had been flooded. I felt a mixture of emotions, as I had psyched myself up and convinced myself that I had the energy and willpower to keep running. It turned out that I wasn't the only one feeling this way, and in the end me and a group of other runners decided to run that day anyway on an unofficial route, so we could still complete as much as possible of the 250 kilometres in five days that we had promised ourselves. Although we didn't quite reach that total, a number of us kept going until we hit over 200 kilometres so that our challenge wasn't cut short. I made the most of the mental energy that I had in me, and it felt like I had earned the reward of the finish line.

Mentally, that experience took me to a completely new level that I hadn't experienced before. I wouldn't say that Sri Lanka was my hardest challenge because they are all difficult in different ways. But it was certainly the most challenging conditions I've ever had to face, and I managed to push through it.

Now, when I am struggling with one of the challenges I take on, I remind myself of the times I almost passed out from the heat. Or the difficulty I had sleeping in such a humid, breezeless climate. Or how dehydration pushed me so far into delirium that when I saw a crocodile only a few feet away, I didn't initially run away (I will share why in a later chapter).

Finishing that ultra-marathon in Sri Lanka was a defining moment for me as it pushed me to the limit. When I was done, I felt such euphoria that I had made it. But the greatest asset it gave me was the ability to know how much I could cope with, and the memories that I have used as motivation for the challenges I have faced since.

Although my experience was extreme, I think this is a lesson we can all apply to every aspect of our lives. If you look at the previous hills you have climbed to get to where you are now, you can dig deeper and find the courage to keep going with the one you're currently facing. The more you do difficult things, the more you believe you are capable of achieving difficult things. You have proof from your own life experiences that you can draw on and use to motivate yourself in tough times. Then, one day, you'll surprise yourself by coasting over the same hurdle without even realizing. When you use your memories as motivation, you will open yourself up to a whole new world of potential.

Lesson 17: You Choose the Energy You Project

Five years after Tano's accident, he had defied all medical expectations through hard work and sheer stubbornness and could walk on crutches. He still occasionally used a wheelchair, but it was spending more and more time folded up and leaning against a wall.

One evening, we went out together to celebrate our friend's birthday at a local pub. I held the door open so Tano could go in first, and he entered the bar with a grin on his face and his crutches in his hands. Cheers greeted him. As I came in behind him, I was nearly knocked over by the swarm of women who had come over to say hello to him. Their response didn't surprise me, because I had witnessed it many times before.

When Tano walks or rolls into a room, he lights it up. His energy radiates outwards, and people are drawn to it because he is so comfortable in his own skin. His attitude is: 'Yeah, I use crutches, and I'm never going to walk the way I once did, but that's just part of my story. I'm also a great father. I'm funny and incredibly ambitious.' I admire him so much for choosing to project himself in that way, and not to let his accident define him. He has taught me that you can decide your own truth, and that it's up to you to choose the energy you project.

Whenever I think about this, it reminds me of kintsugi, which is the Japanese art of mending broken pottery. Instead of throwing a broken plate away or trying to mend a cup handle with 'invisible' glue, they put the pottery back together with a lacquer mixed with powdered gold, silver or platinum. The cracks are highlighted and respected for their history. They are not hidden. They do not signify the end of usefulness or beauty. They are just the next stage of life.

Over the past few years, I have tried to adopt the kintsugi attitude when it comes to my mental health. I've had depression but haven't been depressed for a few years. I struggle with my anxiety, but it is currently manageable. My mindset towards these two things has changed, and I don't feel the need to hide them or pretend they never existed. These gold lines signify the scars from my past and what I have been through. But they also show the restoration work I have done, which ultimately holds me together and makes me who I am.

These mental health conditions are part of me, and I have accepted that they will never fully leave me. But I have learned enough about the way they affect me that I can manage them if they flare up again, and can continue to live a full and fulfilling life. I want to be proud of my history, and not feel that I have to hide it because some people think it's something to be embarrassed about. These conditions are nothing to be ashamed of, and they are just a small part of my formation.

Your kintsugi lines might be different to mine. They

could come from different circumstances or represent other things. Whatever they signify, blend those imperfections with powdered gold, silver or platinum so that you can embrace them and make them a part of your story rather than hiding them away. Once we are comfortable with ourselves and what we have been through, there is an energy shift inside of us and we can project who we are with the kind of positive energy that radiates from Tano. When we are comfortable, we make others comfortable.

By accepting my past struggles, I am now used to talking about them, and because I'm comfortable talking about them, I am asked about them more. By projecting my whole self, scars and all, it enables others to share their whole selves, and changes people's interpretation of what it looks like to live with mental health conditions.

Like Tano, I don't want my challenges to limit me or the standards I expect of myself. My mental health is a part of me, but it does not define me. My struggles are part of my world but not my entire world. I can say this now, with a degree of recovery. In the early days, they were overwhelming, and I tried not to overwhelm others with them. But now, even on the darker days, I know I still have control over the energy that I project and I try to make it as positive as I can.

Lesson 18: Savour the Moment

It is amazing what you can create with a camera tripod, a towel and some stones. My daughter India and I had been happily playing on a pebble beach in Sussex when it began to rain heavily. We were going to get drenched, so I quickly built a makeshift shelter out of what we had around us and she curled up inside. I lay down on my back next to her with my head inside the shelter and the rest of me outside, abandoned to the rain.

My mind went into parent mode, and I said a couple of times that perhaps we should make a dash to the car when the rain lessened. Eventually, she put down the notepad she was happily drawing on and said, 'Why would we want to leave when we're having such a nice time?'

And she was right.

We were having a great time. The part of me that was outside the shelter was already soaked through and couldn't get any wetter. So why disturb this special moment? The rain wasn't deterring her from enjoying what she had right there in front of her. Why should it stop me? So I settled into it, appreciative that at least my head was dry next to her, and I watched as she carried on drawing. We chatted for ages and lost track of time. The rain eased, but we barely noticed. A couple of hours later, we packed up and went and found something to eat, and that memory will stay with me for the rest of my life.

As a parent, perhaps particularly as a single parent, it often feels as though we should maximize every moment we get with our children by taking them on a grand adventure where we end up spending loads of money in an attempt to make them happy. I've been there in the past; there were days when India was younger where I'd take her to do three different things in one day. There might have been stuffed toys and two ice creams bought as well. But that day on the beach was a bit of a wake-up call. I realized that all that other stuff wasn't necessary because she was actually happiest under a towel fort. Now, all my fondest memories of being with India are the simplest ones where we're just having dinner at home or playing in the garden, and it's the same in many other areas of my life. Those simple times of connection are so valuable, and all the money in the world can't buy them.

Children seem to need less than adults think they do. What they want is simplicity and connection and often to be playing outdoors. It's almost like we're moulding them into becoming materialistic. We create this need in them for more things in their lives when they are initially the polar opposite.

So, India and I tend to just hang out together now. We're usually in the Norfolk countryside visiting my dad or up in Lincolnshire with my mum. We go for walks with our dog every day, and often we'll find ourselves at our favourite bench overlooking the beach and sea, in the village I grew up in. We've been there so many times that it feels as if that bench is ours.

I love how the act of sitting quietly in one place outdoors fixes you in the present, and I always savour the special moments where I'm sat peacefully there with her.

When I was partway through the John O'Groats to Land's End wheelchair challenge, my pace setter George and I had just finished scaling an enormous hill and decided to take a break. There was a bench by the side of the road that we wandered over to. Below us was a view of what felt like the entire Lake District. After so many hectic days, sitting there and being present was such a relief and it reminded me of the blissful moments with India.

Often, we just pass those benches by because we are so absorbed in distractions. We are constantly pulled away from our present moment, and we end up living other people's realities rather than our own. When we watch TV, listen to the radio or scroll through social media, we're watching other people's lives – or at least what they want us to see of them. That's why, whenever I go to my and India's bench, I try not to bring my phone unless I want to take a photo. It's a special spot, and it deserves my full attention.

Ask yourself when the last time was that you were

fully present in the moment. You might be very mindful of this and do it twice a day. Or perhaps you haven't had the chance to do it at all recently. If that's the case, maybe it's time to take yourself off and find that bench.

Lesson 19: Keep It Simple

It was the middle of the second day of the ultra-marathon in Sri Lanka, and the intense sun overhead was blasting down on me. I was walking through a muddy paddy field as I no longer had the energy to run. Exhausted and unable to walk in a straight line, I knew I was in trouble. Stumbling along, all I could think about was the heat and how much I needed water. I hadn't seen anyone from our group in hours, and I didn't know who was ahead of me and who was behind. The air was completely still, not even the hint of a breeze, and it felt thick and heavy against my skin. I had stopped sweating a while ago as my body had no more water to give.

I looked around, desperate for shade, but there wasn't a single tree or building in sight. My head was pounding, and my vision began to blur. I was close to passing out, so I sat down to try to compose myself.

The sun was so bright that I squeezed my eyes closed and tried to figure out what to do. Then a rustling noise behind me had me blinking my eyes open. Suddenly I was alert again. Wondering if I had imagined the noise, I turned around and was faced with two teenagers staring down at me. The taller one spoke first, but I didn't understand what he was saying. I asked them if they spoke English, but it was clear they couldn't understand me either.

Before I knew it, they were both scooping water up from a puddle and pouring it over my head. It took a few seconds to understand their reasoning. The water reeked, but I didn't care, as I now knew what they were trying to do – my core temperature had to come down, and the water would help with this. They carried on tipping murky water over me, and gradually my vision began to clear and things became less hazy. I stood up to thank them and nearly fell over. Smiling apologetically, I gestured that I was going to keep on walking. I had to find drinking water. When I turned around to wave to them, they had already gone. I knew I'd never see them again, but I was so grateful they'd spotted me and decided to help. Dousing my body in water had saved me more than they would ever know. It helped me continue for the day and ultimately complete the challenge. They didn't have anything tangible they could give me, but they had given me something more precious than that – their time.

I carried on walking through the paddy field, one foot in front of the other. I don't know how long I had been walking when I glanced up and saw the unmistakable sight of a water station far up ahead. I began a slow jog towards it, my body producing a burst of energy I hadn't known I had. Everything was entirely focused on one thought – *water*. When I got to that small table, I didn't speak to the person behind it and went straight to the water container. Putting my mouth below the tap, I drank until I couldn't physically drink another drop. When I finally stood up, I realized that my clothes were soaked from top to bottom.

If anyone ever asks me what my top five moments are, that taste of water in Sri Lanka is definitely on the list. When we are short of the most essential things we need to survive, our appreciation for them is unquestionable, and they are elevated to the status they should hold. Sri Lanka was the beginning of a journey for me. That gratitude for the simple things in life was absolutely essential for completing my subsequent 76 Marathon challenge. I have so much to be thankful for because of my experience in Sri Lanka. It was fundamental for my future success.

A five-day ultra-marathon in unbearable heat stripped me of everything, and stepping back into a hotel room at the end of it was an alien experience. Everything looked different to how I expected it to appear. When I was able to properly wash five days of dirt from my body and slowly brush my teeth in front of the mirror, I savoured the moment. I was so grateful for those two small acts in a nice bathroom, which before then I had always taken for granted. I had experienced a complete reset, and my appreciation for the simple things in life began again. Later that day, I sat at a table for the first time in five days and ate food with the people I had run with and formed a community with. It reminded me of how important human connection is and how much it had kept me going through that time. Now, I try to wait until I am really hungry before I eat, as the food always tastes so much better and I genuinely value it. That's the problem when everything is so accessible – we often don't appreciate even the food that we have.

Since then, I've been on a mission to simplify so many things in my life so I hold on to the appreciation for the simple things that Sri Lanka taught me. I'm one of the owners of a running training app, Runna, and we recently organized a mental health marathon. What the runners loved about the event was that there was no pressure surrounding it. We didn't have any tracking links or timers. There wasn't any data. We all gathered at the start line, and I started the race by saying, 'This is a run that's different to others. I want you to remember why you are here and who you are running for.' We then counted down together, and it was an emotionally charged moment. When we set off, people ran at their chosen pace, with no expectation of logging stages or beating personal bests. It took the competition element away, and we just enjoyed the connection of our love for running. We kept it simple, and it turned out to be one of our most successful events because of it.

Lesson 20: It's Okay to Put Yourself First Sometimes

'Would this be selfish?' This question is always at the forefront of my mind when I come up with a fresh challenge and begin to fully contemplate it.

At the beginning of 2020, I'd been through a few turbulent years, and going to therapy had helped me to process several things. My relationship had ended with the mother of my child, and the way I was portrayed on a television show wasn't true to the reality of the situation. Because of the way I had been shown, members of the public had come up to me and physically assaulted me in the street. It felt like it had gone too far, and I felt powerless in a situation I hadn't created.

Having been saved by the lifeline of therapy once again, I was reminded of how vital that support was in helping me move forward and get through the dark times. I was lucky that this was an option for me, but I was aware that so many others were not in the same position and I wanted to do something about that. That was when I came up with the idea to run consecutive marathons in every city in the UK to raise money for the Samaritans. They have offices in every city in England, Scotland, Wales and Northern Ireland, and I thought running in each location would help to raise awareness for what they do – to support both them and those who need a lifeline, like I did.

I was so excited about it, thinking about how it could help and inspire so many people. But, as with every decision I make, one person came before everything else – my little girl, India. I always have to weigh up the benefit to the people I am trying to help against the impact my absence will have on her. My challenges have all varied in length, and this one would mean being on the road for two and a half months so it was a really tough call.

My family will always come first in any decision I make, so I spent a long time agonizing over the disruption it might cause versus my desperation to do what was going to fulfil me. While considering whether I could be away for so long, I thought about the people I held as role models in my life. They were all kind and loving, but were also determined and had achieved so much with their time. It made me think that perhaps, as parents, part of being role models for our children is showing them how to be fulfilled and how to chase their dreams and make them happen. I realized that being the best version of myself would enable me to provide more emotional and physical support to those around me. Lifting myself up would help me lift them up too.

It was this thinking that inspired me to proceed with the challenge. At the time, my family weren't keen on the idea, because they were worried about the physical toll it could have on me. Having little experience of running at that time, I reached out to find a coach. I approached Ben Parker, who would later go on to become a big part of my life as one of my business partners in our company, Runna. When I met him for the first time, I pitched him the idea of me running a marathon in every city in the UK. He calmly asked what my running background was and how long I had been doing it for. When I responded saying only a month and my longest run was 10 kilometres, he burst into laughter, only stopping to check if it was a joke. In any ordinary situation, he would have probably turned down the opportunity. But he considered the challenges that I had done previously, such as travelling the length of Britain in a wheelchair. He knew I was ambitious and driven, and my previous achievements were a testament to that. He agreed to become my coach, and the training began to achieve my biggest challenge of all. I wanted to involve India in my training as much as I could, so I would schedule runs with her in a running buggy so she could familiarize herself with what Daddy did.

Then, after a few weeks of training, the world was hit by COVID-19 and the challenge had to be put on hold. All our planning and training stopped overnight and, even three years later, it seemed like one of my greatest ambitions was never going to happen. India was older now, much more aware of time, and I felt that two and a half months was too long to be away from one another.

After returning from running the ultra-marathon in Sri Lanka, I was walking to one of our Runna events early one morning when I came across a young lad's profile on Instagram. He was midway through his challenge of running across Australia to raise money for charity. What he had put himself through and the support his nation had given him really inspired me. Seeing him push himself to his limits to make a difference for others reminded me of my Why, and what I wanted to achieve with the 76 Marathons. If nothing else, the prospect of completing this challenge gave me purpose and made me happy, and this made me the best version of myself — the role model I wanted to be for India. How could I inspire my child to reach for the stars, no matter the hurdles she faced, if I had not done this too? In that moment I knew we had to make it happen. The fire under me was lit again.

Not only did I want to make sure that India knew I was thinking of her while I was away, I also wanted to make her a huge part of the challenge. India travelled up in the camper van with me and the team for part of the journey to the start line of the first marathon. She named the van Elsa Mary-Poppins, which is how we referred to it in our social media posts. India painted my nails so that no matter how far apart we were, whenever she saw any photos or videos, she'd know I was thinking of her. I also arranged for her to visit us on the road in different cities, and it all became part of the adventure for her. I loved those days. I would sit in the camper van, sore and broken, and watch my little girl be part of the team and get stuck in, either cleaning up after us or adding to the mess. On the days she was away, we would regularly FaceTime. Looking back on it, it worked out so well.

Some people might think that spending time on your own goals is selfish, but sometimes you have to make difficult, unconventional decisions to be true to who you really are. Never in a million years did I see myself becoming someone who does challenges in wheelchairs and runs across countries, but I've found myself here. I hope that what I've done will have a positive impact on the world, not just in terms of mental health awareness but my relationship with India too.

We often praise people for their selflessness, for how they put everyone else first or give others the clothes off their back. This is wonderful but, when it comes to parenting, I don't believe that self-sacrifice, where we give up our whole lives to ensure our children always come first, is necessarily the best thing for them. If we want to inspire our children and show them a world full of possibility, we might need to do that by putting ourselves first occasionally. Sometimes bold decisions are the hardest to make, but ultimately they can provide the most transformative outcomes.

This isn't just about parents sacrificing their dreams for their children, however. If we consistently put someone else's day-to-day needs before our own lifetime dreams or goals, there is likely to be an imbalance, and it might have a long-term detrimental effect. If we're always focused on others, we're distracted from ourselves.

You can become a role model to anyone who comes

into your life, and even those who never meet you in person. Therefore, it's your decision what type of role model you want to be. If I want my daughter to inherit a limitless mindset and believe that anything is possible, she has to be able to look at her closest role models and see that belief in them. I am proud to be one of those people. By doing these challenges, I hope they will help her to have faith in herself.

Lesson 21: There is No Such Thing as the Perfect Time

We were a few weeks into the first lockdown of COVID-19, and my training for the 76 Marathons had been stopped in its tracks. I was living by myself, hadn't seen my friends or family for weeks and had very little to fill the time, when I received a telephone call from the charity Campaign Against Living Miserably (CALM), who I had been in contact with about potentially supporting them. They told me they had received a 38 per cent increase in telephone calls since the beginning of lockdown, from people struggling with mental illness. This affected me deeply, and I looked around my house and thought about what I could do to help.

Later that day, I had an idea that wouldn't leave me, and I ended up measuring my tiny patio at 1 a.m. in the morning to see if what I had come up with was possible.

The following day, I called my coach and told him I wanted to run five marathons around my fourteen-foot patio in five days. The measurements I had taken in the early hours of the morning confirmed that to reach one mile I would have to run eighty loops. Therefore, I would have to run approximately 2,096 laps of my patio every day for five days to complete the challenge. My coach thought it was a great idea, but was concerned about the reality of the impact it would have on my body.

Undeterred, I spoke to several other people about it. The overwhelming verdict was that it would take a considerable toll on my body, and I should perhaps think about doing something else. Running consecutive tight loops would put repeated pressure on the same parts of my body and could easily cause an injury. There was also an increased risk because at this point I had only been training for the 76 Marathons for a few months.

Was I properly prepared to do this? Absolutely not. But I also knew there would never be the 'perfect' time for it.

As it turned out, it was absolutely the perfect moment for me to do it. Even though it seemed like the craziest idea because I had never run consecutive marathons before and a tiny patio was not an ideal place to do this, it struck a chord with many people sitting at home with not much to do. They needed something to root for, and I wanted to raise money and awareness for the work CALM was doing. After three days, I exceeded my target of raising £2,000. Because of this and entirely on the spur of the moment, I decided to extend the challenge and run six marathons in five days. In the end, the challenge raised over £24,000. Even if you might not think you are ready to do something, sometimes the stars align to create a perfect moment and you just have to run with it (not literally, although I did).

Two weeks later, I set myself a further challenge of

running around the same patio for twenty-four hours straight. I had got the bug for it, perhaps because we were still in lockdown, and I couldn't get the idea out of my head to run around it for a whole day without stopping. I now knew that it was a pretty ideal place to run as I had all the facilities I needed on hand. However, people usually take months to prepare for their first 24-hour race, and they certainly don't do it two weeks after their first consecutive marathons. But I knew the timing was right so I did it, and I raised a further £22,500 for CALM.

The stars were also aligned when I eventually ran the 76 consecutive marathons three years later. Despite feeling like it was never going to happen, it caught the public's attention, and many people joined in and ran with me, and we ended up raising close to £400,000 for the Samaritans.

There are so many factors to consider when it comes to big decisions – many of which are outside our control and will never be in our control – so sometimes we need to take a leap of faith. If we delay by waiting for the perfect time, we justify the rationale for not doing something and deny ourselves from experiencing a perfect moment. Instead, we need to look at the long-term picture, weigh up the pros and cons of our decision, and decide if it's fear that is holding us back or a legitimate reason. There will never be a perfect time to do something, as we cannot predict what will happen in the future. I could have waited for India to be much older to do the 76 Marathons, but by then, I might have been struggling with an injury or facing countless unimaginable obstacles. Also, the challenge's purpose was to highlight the rise of mental illness and lack of support. By waiting years to do this, there would be so many people we potentially could have helped and didn't. On a purely personal level, I knew it was a great idea and would have kicked myself if I was the one to have come up with it but someone else completed it.

It wasn't the perfect time to find out that I was going to be a dad three weeks after I had separated from India's mum. No one would see that as ideal, but walking away was never an option, so I adapted. And a lifetime of perfect moments came from that experience. I'm so thankful for the person I've become because of India and the memories we have made together.

Looking back at every challenge I've gone into, I've never been fully prepared. I don't think it's possible to ever feel fully prepared for the significant moments in life. Nothing can prepare you for the unknown – becoming a parent, quitting a job or moving somewhere new. There has to be a degree of preparation, of course, but there is a fine line between being prepared and waiting for the perfect time that will never come.

It's easy to procrastinate and put something off, even if it's something we're excited about, for fear of the outcome. Our instinct is to stay safe and not take the risk. We can put up hurdles to stop ourselves from doing something or to justify the delay, but if we were the ones to put up those hurdles, we also have the power to pull them down.

Lesson 22: You Get More from the Hard Things in Life

Towards the end of the John O'Groats to Land's End challenge, we had fallen seriously behind. On average, we had been doing around 50 miles each day, but our timings had slipped. Down in Cornwall, the roads were wet and slippery, which was a nightmare to navigate in a wheelchair. Throughout the challenge to that point, I hadn't flipped my wheelchair once and had managed to remain upright the entire time. Then I fell out of my wheelchair four or five times in three days, which was painful and demoralizing. On a couple of occasions, it was also quite terrifying.

There can be a feeling of absolute terror when you flip a wheelchair and your legs are strapped in. When you trip while running, you have the chance to right yourself. But in a wheelchair, when you hit a stone or a divot, or clip a car, you automatically lose control – and unfortunately the odds of you staying upright are very much stacked against you. There is very little you can do to break your fall in a wheelchair. And not only are you falling, but you're attached to the wheelchair – something heavy enough to break bones. While I was training in London, I learned that many wheelchair users suffer PTSD after falls from or in their wheelchairs, which was something I had never even considered before.

By 5 p.m. on the penultimate day, we had fallen way behind and had only covered 23 miles. We'd had a great morning together and spirits were high, but we had somehow gone way off schedule. The impact this would have on the following day would be huge. We had no choice but to push on.

It was pitch-black when we reached the 40-mile mark, and I was a broken man. There were no streetlights, as we were in such a remote area, and the only illumination came from the headlights of the support car. Our pace was excruciatingly slow from the combination of the gradients of the hills and the limited light, and we were still 10 miles short of where we needed to be. My pace setter George was mentally exhausted, so he swapped with Kris King, who came and walked with me. I didn't begrudge George that; it just showed how challenging our situation was.

We could have stopped for the day, but we didn't. What I was doing was hard, but I wouldn't let myself take the easy way out. For weeks we had been picturing the final day of the challenge, and it was so close now. All of our friends and family would be travelling down to meet us, and we wanted to finish the challenge around lunchtime so we could spend the afternoon celebrating with them. We didn't want to roll in late in the afternoon. India would be there with my parents, and I was desperate to spend some proper time with her. I knew

I would get more out of continuing with the hard thing I was doing rather than going with the easy option.

So we carried on and eventually covered the last 10 miles late in the evening, knowing all the way that we'd have to get up at 4 a.m. to complete the challenge in time. That night, I climbed into bed, still soaked in sweat, for four hours of sleep.

Hard things are a must in life. Many people hate the following line, but I really do believe that what doesn't kill you makes you stronger. Having come close to taking my own life because of my mental health conditions, I feel so passionate about that saying. I truly believe that when my depression and anxiety didn't kill me, they made me stronger. They propelled me to where I am now, and gave me the purpose of making it more acceptable for people to talk about their own mental health struggles, and helping them find strength in their vulnerability like I did. The gain from finding that purpose has ultimately led to a life of fulfilment for me.

When we can accept that we are going to face hardships, we stand a better chance of learning from them. They can even become our fuel if we look at them the right way.

Through my work, I am privileged to meet many inspiring people such as activists, athletes, public speakers, authors and entrepreneurs. So many of them have used their hardships to spur them into action. They have utilized their past – what they have faced and overcome – to provide momentum for the future. As they achieve more, their strength and their resilience have increased, and they gain the experience that helps them navigate any further difficult situations that come their way. They deal with whatever comes up in whatever capacity they can.

Too often, we idolize these individuals. We believe they have led charmed lives, which has enabled them to succeed. When in fact their experiences are often the opposite, and what they have gained from the challenges they've faced are resilience, determination and purpose. This is a choice that we can make for ourselves as well. Will we see our hardships as holding us back, or can we use them to propel us forward?

Lesson 23: Don't Do Something to Prove Someone Wrong – Do It to Prove Yourself Right

India and I were staying with my dad for a few days in Norfolk. We had all been holed up together for a while, and I wanted to get out of the house for an hour. India needed batteries for one of her toys, so this seemed the perfect reason to take my motorbike to the nearest town to buy them for her. When I briefly mentioned my plan to my dad, he told me it was going to rain and I shouldn't ride my motorbike. This statement seems simple enough, but it followed several days of my dad's unsolicited advice in various areas of my life. Something in me snapped, and I found myself telling him that I was thirty-three years old, and if I wanted to ride my bike, I would.

I hugged India goodbye and explained I'd be back soon with batteries. My dad shouted after me again that it was going to rain, and I ignored him. He'd been telling me what to do for the past three days, and I was tired of it. I wasn't twelve; I could make simple decisions (and complex ones) for myself. I made them all the time, and I hadn't done too badly.

Starting up my bike, I eased it out of the driveway.

Opening up the throttle, I enjoyed riding along the quiet country lanes.

What happened next? It began to chuck it down.

Heavy rain isn't pleasant to ride in or very safe, so I slowed down and found a quiet place to turn around and return home. When I opened the door, my dad was standing in the hallway. He took one look at me, soaked to the skin, and cracked up. I put my hands up and said, 'I'm sorry. You were one hundred per cent right. I got soaked.' We were laughing about it for the rest of the evening.

When we do something to prove to someone else that they're wrong, we're immediately setting ourselves up for failure. Letting our ego take priority will always be to our detriment. It will cloud our judgement and prevent us from considering all the factors we need to take into account (like whether there are rain clouds in the sky) and force us to push on regardless. The focus shifts from doing something we enjoy for ourselves to something we must complete despite our best interests.

This is a small example, but I have pursued things for the wrong reason several times before. The four-minute-mile attempt came from wanting to show the doubters they were wrong. Inevitably, this wasn't particularly successful because the intention behind it didn't come from a genuine place. But when I subsequently helped set up a running app, Runna, with its two co-founders, Ben Parker and Dom Maskell, I finally had the right intentions. It has been hugely successful because I wasn't doing it to prove anyone wrong. I was doing it because I believed in it to my very core. I look back on the moment that I shared my idea with Ben on the Barnes running track and was elated to hear that he and Dom had had similar conversations and shared my vision for an app that changed the face of running. I instinctively knew it was a great idea and wanted to prove to myself that what I thought was correct. That is a place of positivity. That is a place from which you can set off and succeed.

Lesson 24: Your Relationships Can Impact Your Mental Health

The start of my parents' marriage could have been taken straight from a romance-film script. My dad came from absolute poverty in Ballymena in Northern Ireland, while my mum came from a much more secure background. But they crossed this divide and were married within four weeks of meeting each other.

My mum's family wouldn't accept the marriage, so my parents set off by themselves. Their first house was a one-up, one-down. They had an ironing board for a table and only one stool. When they ate dinner together, my mum would sit on the stool and my dad on the floor. Against all odds, they built an empire together and were married for thirty years. Boy and girl meet, and live happily ever after. That's how the story goes, right?

But what these types of films often fail to properly explore is the experiences someone has growing up and how this shapes them. My dad came from poverty, which was tough enough as it was, but he also had a difficult home life as well. He was from a large family, with six children in a small house, so he grew up sharing a bed with his sisters. Other than basic clothes and food, his parents couldn't afford to buy him anything growing up. He often tells the story of how delighted he was when he found a bike meant for scrap in the street; it didn't even have any tyres or brakes but he found some green paint and used a stick to cover up the rust with it. The bike must have looked like a right mess, but he was so happy to ride it around on the metal rims. When telling me this story, he laughed about how sparks would fly up as he cycled it around on the cobbles. He also told me about how his parents could barely afford shoes that fitted him, let alone the ones all the other children had with spikes in them that they needed for sport, and so he would stuff his shoes full of newspaper and then put pins through the soles so he could compete in the long jump at school.

My grandfather, his dad, had been a successful businessman who'd owned several butcher's shops but was called away to fight in the Second World War and returned a changed man. He came back to his business in tatters and with little opportunity to find work and provide for his family. The pressure of supporting his family while dealing with the trauma of what he'd been through in the war became too much, and ultimately was his undoing. Alcohol became his coping mechanism, and this subsequently impacted my dad and his siblings. It sounded like the more pressure he was under to support his family, the more he turned to drink, and it became a vicious cycle which resulted in my dad being kicked out of the house on a couple of occasions, at the ages of just nine and twelve. I think about my gorgeous little girl now and I can't imagine how traumatizing that must have been for such a young child to go through.

Finding himself on the streets in Northern Ireland in the 1950s, there was a lot of violence all around him and he saw some terrible things. Apparently, where he was from, only Catholics could learn to box, so he pretended to be Catholic so he could learn how to defend himself.

My dad's refuge was his mum, who he adored. She was one of those unsung women who should be recognized for what she did for her family. She was full of love, and had very little materially but was grateful for everything she had. She did her very best to shield her children from the harshness of the world, but she couldn't always protect them from their own father.

My dad's experiences and his relationship with my grandfather definitely shaped him. They made him determined, and a survivor. He used them to push through adversity and later build a successful business alongside my mum. When I think about what my dad went through, it makes me so grateful for being brought up by two parents who loved me and, most importantly, knew how to show me love. It is such a shame that my mum and dad didn't get their fairy-tale ending and live happily ever after. When I look at their marriage, I often think about how their story ended and what our lives would be like now if those traumas and issues had been approached differently.

The type of trauma my dad faced can pass down through generations. But my dad made sure that my sister and I knew we were loved, which wasn't the legacy his own father had left. He also supported our dreams and goals and made so many sacrifices for us, driving us endless miles to whichever training session we had that week as children – the kind of support he never received from his own father when he was growing up. Unlike his dad, even when he found himself in a heart-breaking situation, he always put us first. He gave me a job as a labourer when I needed one at my lowest time, and he also threatened to fire me from that job if I didn't take the leap and accept my first opportunity to be on a TV show.

Our relationships form a large part of our environment, if not the most crucial part. In our younger years, the relationships we have with people at home, particularly our parents, shape our outlook. When we get older, relationships with friends or a partner will begin to play a more significant role. Living with someone and spending time with them on a daily basis literally shapes your existence. That is why it is so important to be alert to the effect a relationship has on your mental health and also whether the person supports you in achieving your goals and ambitions.

I am very aware of how relationships can impact mental health. My anxiety can affect my mood, but I know that it isn't always obvious to someone else, which can cause miscommunication and conflict. I now know that it's important to be around people who are mindful of that and who have the empathy and maturity to understand that when I'm quiet it's not because of something they have done. Instead, it's because of something I am going through. We don't need to make a big deal of it, and I will quietly work through my funk and then be back to my usual chatty self.

While running the 76 Marathons, I spoke to someone who had decided to stop drinking as they had realized how their approach to alcohol was holding them back. They had been in a relationship for five years, and their partner wasn't ready to cut back and had even tried to deter them from doing it. The two of them had found themselves on different paths and couldn't find the bridge between them, so they'd separated. Our relationships shape our environment, and our environment either helps or hinders our journey.

Just as our relationships can hold us back, they can also provide huge amounts of support. I'll never forget a message I received from a woman on social media who was worried about her boyfriend. She told me her partner was really struggling and had become very emotional, which wasn't like him. He was intently focused on his career, but his employer kept moving the goalposts and he felt lost. She wanted to know if I, as a mental health advocate, had any advice for him. In the end, I met with him, and we chatted about his situation. After we had spoken about his work, I told him that the lesson I would take from this experience was that he had an absolute diamond of a girlfriend and he should do everything he could to keep her in his life. For her to reach out to me because she was concerned for him showed her commitment and love, which needed to be recognized.

Looking after your mental health in relationships is a careful balance of give and take. You have to be alert to the impact a relationship has on you. But equally, you have to consider how you impact those around you, something we will cover in the next chapter.

Lesson 25: Your Relationships are There to Support but Not Fix Your Problems

When I was approached for advice by the girlfriend of someone struggling with their mental health, as described in the last chapter, it was a true testament to her love and compassion for her partner. She showed empathy and understanding, but how her boyfriend responded to this also helped to determine the course of their relationship.

She did the groundwork to support her vulnerable partner, and when he heard about this, he had a choice to make. He could acknowledge the problem and do something about it, or ignore it and continue with the cycle he was in. He decided to reciprocate her kindness and care by putting the work in from his end. He searched for something outside of his career to focus on and give him purpose. He spent some of his free time training for a Tough Mudder, which is a challenging running event with various obstacles to face. The combination of the endorphin-boosting exercise and having something to think about outside of his stress-inducing work helped his mental well-being. His newfound purpose was admirable, and his girlfriend felt closer to him in response. She recognized she was in a relationship with a man who tackled his problems head-on. Their actions created a firm foundation of mutual respect, which is essential for all long-term relationships.

I don't think anyone with any empathy would say that having a mental health condition or poor mental well-being is easy. But it's not always easy being in a relationship with someone going through this either. There are two people in a relationship, and both need empathy and love from their partner. We show our strength by being open about what we are feeling and experiencing. However, this is just part of it; we also have to hear and acknowledge what our partner is going through as well. What we are experiencing will probably impact them, which needs to be recognized.

The solution isn't to just talk about ourselves and our problems all the time, especially if we're not doing anything to improve them. People will invest in us the amount we invest in ourselves. So, if we're constantly going through this negative cycle and there doesn't seem to be any desire to rectify the situation, people are unlikely to have unending patience and compassion. If those around us suggest constructive ideas but we ignore them all, we might begin to be viewed as a lost cause.

It's a two-way street, and the lines of communication need to be open in both directions. If those lines need reopening, therapy can help. Therapy can be such a godsend in these situations – as long as you have the right therapist. Sometimes when a neutral party rephrases an idea you have been trying to explain, the other person can suddenly absorb it and there is progression in a situation that previously felt unsolvable.

People with mental health struggles or addictions can react to their individual situation in a variety of ways, and many of them are completely valid. It might take a bit of time for them to tackle the problem, or they might address it immediately. They could prefer loads of support or hardly any, therapy or no therapy, medication or none. People are different, and therefore there are a variety of possible approaches. What isn't a valid way of dealing with issues is to be aggressive, controlling or overly dramatic. That's inexcusable, and we can't use a condition to try to excuse that behaviour. No diagnosis gives us permission to be abusive.

When it comes to relationships in general, the synergy has to be right. The balance of how much we can give and take must work in alignment with the partner we have. So many people end up with a partner who isn't right for them. That doesn't make either of them a bad person; it's just a case of two good people not being the right fit for each other. If you're in a relationship where the fit isn't right, and you suspect it's much harder than it should be, nobody is at fault or in the wrong. You're just incompatible. And if you're unsuited, you'll probably wear each other down because you're constantly grating on each other.

You need someone you're mentally aligned with because then the relationship will run more smoothly. It will be easier, which means that when inevitable hardships or struggles happen, you're in a stronger position to face them together.

Lesson 26: The Mind–Body Connection is Powerful

When I began training for marathons, I realized that when you have been exercising for several hours, you inevitably reach a point where you want to give up. I'd start thinking about all the valid excuses I could use to duck out, such as an ache in my leg, or tell myself that I could catch up on the mileage the next day or try again another time. This is usually the mind playing tricks on us, because our bodies are powerful and designed for survival – and can continue for much longer and deal with much more than we might initially realize.

The key to any test of endurance is to push through this barrier, because once you do, your mind will realize how much your body can cope with. You might even enter that beautiful state of flow where everything seems possible and you don't even know why you wanted to stop.

There is a yin and yang element to this, as the mind and body are opposite but interconnected forces that send messages to each other. The mind controls the body, and we are all aware of this, but the body also sends signals back to the brain, which we might often ignore. If you can get the two to connect, this ultimately delivers the best outcome.

I learned how to find this balance years ago, and it was incredible to finally learn which signals to listen to and which ones I could push past, and that has stayed with me ever since – and I think it is something we can all benefit from.

When we know how the body and mind communicate, it can be difficult to analyse how we are really feeling and connect with the state of our physical or mental health – we are either too busy to pay attention to the warning signals or won't know what signs to look out for. But the body will often subtly alert us if something, either physically or mentally, isn't right. I know that if I'm not in a good place mentally or I am really stressed or overworked, my skin condition – psoriasis – will flare up again. It's a clear sign that I need to slow down, take care of myself, and relieve some of the pressure I'm under if I can.

This is because my body is an expression of my mindset, and this applies to my physical fitness too. When I am in shape, my mental health is much better. This is partly because I have a more positive outlook when I feel physically healthy. But it is also because when I'm happier, I am more proactive and motivated to train, which leads me to exercise more and, consequently, I feel more optimistic. It's a cycle where my body and my mind feed into each other and bring about the best outcome. As opposed to other times in my life, when I suffer a drop in mood and have a worse outlook on myself and my life, simply because I'm not exercising.

I know that being in shape is good for my mental health on many levels, but this can be misconstrued as vanity. I don't go to the gym because I want a six-pack. I do it because it helps me fulfil my purpose of completing these challenges and because exercise makes me feel good and keeps me fit and strong. It's not about aesthetics, it's about how it makes me feel.

We all come in different shapes and sizes so there's no point in aiming to look the same as anyone else. It's about learning to listen to your body and mind so that you can feel happy in your own skin each day. But in order to enjoy the happiness it brings for as long as possible and have the longest life you can, it's important to exercise and eat a balanced diet for the health benefits they both bring. It can be hard for your brain to overrule your body and force yourself to go outside into the cold to face the gym or go on a run, but if there is something telling you that you will feel better for it then you should listen to those powerful signals. This isn't to alter how you appear on the outside, but for what it does for you on the inside, and to get the best out of both your body and your mind.

Lesson 27: Don't Take
Your Body for Granted

In 2021, I had set myself my biggest challenge to date, which was to run a marathon in each country in the UK within twenty-four hours. Run 4 Nations combined having to run more than 168 kilometres in a single day and fit in travelling between the four countries as well. The stakes were high, and the pressure was on. Logistically, it was incredibly tricky, as between marathons the team would have to travel to a different country, and the only way we could do this within the set time was by helicopter. We started with a marathon in Northern Ireland and then took a helicopter to Scotland, where I ran the next one that led me down into England, where I ran the third. We then took a helicopter to Wales, where I completed the last marathon.

Looking back at it, I didn't prepare or train in the way that I would do now, and my body paid the price. During the second marathon, in Scotland, I began limping and I later found out that the ligaments in my knee, calf and foot were damaged. The pain grew so bad that I was projectile-vomiting into a carrier bag, and by the fourth marathon, in Wales, I didn't know how I would be able to run anymore as I could barely walk. But my team strapped my leg up, the adrenaline kicked in, and the fluidity came back to my running. From then on, it was just a case of praying that my body would stay together for as long as possible.

Despite these injuries, my body did keep going. It was my first real experience of what the body is capable of under extreme pressure. I was completely in awe of what it could do, and incredibly grateful for how resilient it was. From this came a change to my career, which has enabled me to meet the most remarkable people from around the world. It's allowed me to inspire others to go further and fulfil their own dreams and goals.

Before I did this challenge it was very hard for me to appreciate my body. I could be critical of it and didn't really understand what I had. The challenge brought about an epiphany that would be cemented by my future challenges and the people I met who were doing similar challenges or had faced life-changing illnesses or injuries. The fact that our bodies keep going despite what happens to them is incredible, and they should be respected for that. When I did Run 4 Nations, I didn't have the right nutrition, wasn't getting enough sleep and my training wasn't ideal, yet still my body carried me through. It's not something I would repeat in the same way because it could easily have led to a permanent injury, but I now knew what my body would be capable of with the right food and training.

Through my experience of these challenges, and all the mistakes I've made over the past six years, I've really learned to be grateful for my body and what it does for me. It's easy to take this for granted, but we have to consider what we want to accomplish in life, how far we wish to go, how long for and whether the way we are treating our bodies will help us accomplish that. How do we want to feel while we're doing it? Have we damaged our bodies, and can the damage be rectified? I'm not talking about people who have sustained the worst medical conditions completely outside their control, but the people who have a functioning body and mind but aren't taking care of them. Often this comes down to not having an appreciation or love for ourselves or our bodies – but this attitude can be changed, and I've done it myself.

We are told that we should be 'living our best life', which can be taken as an encouragement to throw caution to the wind. But what it actually means is often distorted. It's not about taking loads of drugs, drinking excessively, smoking, or eating everything we can lay our hands on. And because the negative consequences are not always immediately noticeable, we don't realize the long-term mental and physical damage we're doing. There are many other things we can focus our energy on that don't harm the body. I would say that 'living our best life' is living a fulfilled one and, crucially, a long one, which we will only achieve if we look after ourselves.

Even when people get involved in something that is outwardly healthy, such as fitness, it can still be destructive if they approach it with the wrong mindset. And the body will pay the price, because the body and mind are connected. When I was first taking on challenges, I would throw myself into one after another. I see this same pattern in other people now, and I think there is a problem with it because they are not enjoying it or feeling fulfilled. Often, the people who take on extreme challenge after extreme challenge are trying to fill a void, rather than have a positive impact. Their bodies will keep on going to complete breaking point, because it's only when the mind is fatigued and exhausted that the body will shut down.

We each need to consider the decisions we are making for our body, and what will benefit it and what won't. This isn't about vanity or appearance; we should all love our bodies regardless of their shape or size. But there are choices we can make to help the body function well, and we need to treat it with respect, just as we would if it was another person. After all, it is the most important tool we have been gifted to enable us to live a prosperous life.

Lesson 28: Acknowledge Your Greatness

I believe that I am great.

Before you write me off as completely full of myself, I firmly believe that we should all say this to ourselves more often. Everyone is great in their own unique way. We all contribute something to the world, but most of us lose sight of our own value over time. Our identity is shaped by what we hear and think about ourselves, so we need to hear positive affirmations about ourselves to build our confidence. If we say negative things about ourselves to others, we will begin to believe them, and ultimately, they will limit us. Self-doubt will take over, and we won't put ourselves out there, take risks or set ourselves up for success.

There is nothing wrong with believing in yourself and acknowledging the great things about who you are. It's actually vital if you want to achieve anything in life. This kind of appreciation shouldn't be misinterpreted as arrogance or narcissism. It's just you telling yourself something true and believing it. The more you say it, the more you will begin to believe it. If you also back it up with evidence of what you have achieved in the past and against what odds, then you really will create true confidence in your own abilities. Alternatively, if you go into something unable to appreciate yourself, nerves will take over and the cracks will begin to show. Once that happens, there is less chance of success, because either you won't inspire others to believe in what you're doing, or you'll talk yourself out of it.

I don't think I am an extraordinary runner, but by surrounding myself with exceptional people, I can then go on to do exceptional things. To prepare for the 76 Marathons, I needed to do a lot of strength and conditioning work. I could have gone to the gym and done that on my own, but I chose not to. Instead, I had my trainer, Nick, with me, as he is one of the exceptional people I surround myself with, which gives me an edge. His work is the difference between me and the next person. I knew that to run the 76 Marathons, I would need someone who was a great runner, was invested in the meaning behind the challenge as much as I was, and had a determined mindset. An added bonus would be if they had the organizational skills I sometimes need help with. That's one of the reasons I asked Chris Taylor to join the challenge as my coach and team leader, as I knew he would be a huge asset to me and the rest of the team. All the team members I work with are exceptional at what they do and elevate me to where I need to be.

It is easy to shy away from spending time around people who are better than us at what we want to achieve – to see them as competitors. But we shouldn't be too afraid or proud to be around these people. Rather than falling into that trap, we should learn from them, ask questions, and use their knowledge to level up our skills. Someone else's greatness doesn't detract from your own; in fact it can make you greater.

It is important to recognize where our greatness comes from. For me, I think it is the ability to connect with people, so I lean into this by surrounding myself with extraordinary people. It is this that enables me to achieve difficult things, not my ability alone. For you, it might be something you are studying, a passion you've had from a young age, a rare skill, or a unique perspective that has given you immense drive. Wherever it comes from, you need to recognize what makes you special so you can encourage more of it rather than allowing it to fade away.

When you embrace your talents and see your progression, it won't feel as weird to say to yourself that you're great. Finally, you'll start to believe it.

Lesson 29: Don't Ignore Your Weaknesses

I was panicking, scrolling through my emails again for what felt like the hundredth time. I was being chased by someone for a contract I'd been meant to sign three weeks ago, but I was certain I hadn't received it. The search function hadn't brought anything up, but I carried on scrolling through the messages, the email subject lines blurring together as my dyslexic brain struggled to make head or tail of what I was looking at. Suddenly I saw it: the email from DocuSign was on the fourth page, and I'd missed it. I pulled it up and began to read through it; my undiagnosed ADHD mind desperately wanting to bounce off and think about something else.

In the last chapter, we covered the benefits of recognizing that we're great. But this is not the same as thinking we're great at everything, because the reality is that no one can be. Just as we should accept our natural talents, I think it's equally important to accept our weaknesses, rather than fighting against them.

As the story above demonstrates, one of mine is that I'm not very organized. I try to be, but I sometimes unintentionally miss an email or am late for a meeting. I have a calendar on my phone and check it regularly, but occasionally I'll miss out on the crucial step of putting an appointment into my calendar. I'll be about to put one in, get distracted, and the thought won't enter my head again until someone is messaging me about whether I can still make a call that started five minutes ago. It's not my ego that does this or a sign of me not valuing the other person's time. It is simply how my mind works, as I don't always make all the links between A, B and C to ensure something happens. I'll be between A and B, and get distracted by a new idea, P, which is much further down the line.

This always used to hold me back and sometimes I would get annoyed with myself, but then I realized that my struggle to focus meant that I also had a creative mind and could sometimes pre-empt circumstances. I decided then to embrace this difference rather than push against it.

Now, whenever I go into challenges, I try to create a plan that works with my weaknesses. I love running and connecting with people, but I can get distracted when training in the gym or on the track. When I have a day like that ahead of me, I will look at the plan that has been prepared for me and think, 'I don't want to follow this today.' My mind is like a ping-pong ball, and I'll want to go off and do some extra sets on something else. I have learned to combat this by having my strength and conditioning coach, Nick, with me. We work really well together because he understands my mechanics, both mentally and physically. I realized that to get the best out of me when I train, I must enjoy it. I need the balance of focus and fun, and Nick fulfils that every time I step into the gym. I love training with him, so I push myself harder and follow the plan he has made. It's the same with my running coach, Chris. Both of them know how to elevate me by working with my weaknesses.

Everyone has different ways of approaching things, especially when you think about neurodivergent brains (those with autism, dyslexia and ADHD, to name a few) and neurotypical brains, so when we acknowledge the things that we're good at and not so good at, it enables us to elevate each other to new heights. Rather than being proud and trying to do everything ourselves, we can get so much further if we work as part of a team. When it comes to our running training app, Runna, I know that my two business partners are exceptional guys in completely different ways, and they also have completely different weaknesses. Ben's unbelievable determination and Dom's intelligence and capabilities are a winning combination. Having worked together for a couple of years we now know how to complement each other's skill sets. When I first entered that office, I was the least qualified person there. I've never been to university; I have one A-level and only three GCSEs and didn't know how to use a spreadsheet or create a presentation. But I knew that if I went into a room, I could connect with people on a level like no other. I can get the best out of people because I genuinely love learning about them and figuring out what inspires them. I've always known that you get the best out of people through the connection you make with them, not from the numbers you give them.

Instead of ignoring my weaknesses or feeling constrained by them, I try to improve them where I can or surround myself with people who can help me level up. At Runna, I made it clear to Ben and Dom where my weaknesses were, so they were aware of them, while also highlighting my strengths. Taking this open approach meant there were no surprises, and I also decided to work hard to improve where I could. I've learned about spreadsheets and check my diary several times a day. I'm also pretty amazing at Canva now, as I needed to learn how to use it if I wanted to become the Presentation King. We need to be proud of the small things we learn and celebrate them, because that sets the tone for others celebrating their own wins.

I have no formal qualifications, and six years ago I used to dodge my roommate's request for me to join him on a run. Now I am a co-owner of a running app and I couldn't imagine my life without running. I also view the fact that I haven't always been a runner as a benefit. I still remember when I didn't run, and what helped in the early days to motivate me and build the habit of running until it was something I loved.

Too many people stop themselves from doing things in life because, on paper, it doesn't make sense. They think they're underqualified, inexperienced or don't have the right skills or talents. But the thing is, you don't need to have *all* the necessary skills to do something. If you're aware of where your areas of weakness are, you can keep on learning and improve your skills by surrounding yourself with people who help or complement you in those areas.

We should always recognize our strengths, but also our weaknesses – because there is always the option to improve them.

Lesson 30: You're Never Too Old for a Snowball Fight

Weather extremes always make marathons twice as hard. The baking sun can raise your heart rate to dangerous levels, and gusts of wind can quite literally hold you back. During the marathon in Lisburn, the thirteenth of the 76 Marathons challenge, we faced compacted snow, which can have you on your knees in a second. It had been minus-five degrees the previous night and snowing in Northern Ireland for a whole day. By the morning, the snow had finally stopped, but it was still freezing cold and dangerously slippery in places.

We had two ways of approaching this situation we found ourselves in. We could either let it bring our energy down and cast a shadow over the day, or try to make the best of it. Chris was running ahead of me when I couldn't resist the temptation any longer. I bent down, scooped up some snow, made it into a ball, and launched it at his head. Bullseye. He stopped for a moment before swinging around, scooping up his own snowball for revenge. We pelted each other for ten minutes before realizing we still had a marathon to run. So, we made up a game where the one in front would throw snowballs at the person behind without looking, and the person at the back couldn't dodge out of the way to avoid them. Chris and I ran like this for two hours, taking turns to be the target. We both got snowballs straight in the face a few times and just had to hold ourselves still as we watched them arc towards us. That one game turned around our approach to what could have been a pretty shocking marathon in ice-cold temperatures with slippery ground to cover. That first snowball led to two hours of distraction and fun.

We were two men in their thirties lobbing snowballs at each other to pass the time. Some people might view it as a bit immature, but I like to view it as seeing the joy in life. As we get older, we can decide to become more worn down by the world and our experiences of it, or we can try to hold on tightly to that brilliant, joyful optimism we had as children.

Growing up, so many of us feel invincible, and we skip through life in our pursuit of adventure and fun. It is only as we get older and face bigger knock-backs that we start to get a sense of limitations. Left unchallenged, we can carry those limitations with us into adulthood and let them dictate what we do. But we can also choose to look past them and carry our natural optimism into our older bodies if we choose to. We can view the world with a bit of joy and lightness, just as children do who don't see all the can'ts and shouldn'ts. Kids don't view the weather as a limitation that will stop their day. Instead, they just put on their boots and go outside and play. I never want to lose that ability to get to the most positive outcome in any situation, and I've found that slowing down to enjoy the moment helps to do this.

We live in a time where we take a very hurried approach to everything. The pace is intense, which affects our mindset and what we take from our experiences. When we slow down to enjoy a moment and play with it, it triggers all those emotions we enjoyed as children.

Of course, many situations call for maturity, but certainly not all of them. Sometimes, we need to embrace the adult version of ourselves, and sometimes our inner child. Because there is still a small child in each of us, and we can reconnect with them by allowing them to come out and play.

Lesson 31: We Learn Through Making Mistakes

It was November, and I was standing in the hallway of my dad's house in Norfolk, waiting for India. We were about to go for a walk, as our dog needed to get outside even on a cold, cloudy morning. India came down the stairs wearing a purple net skirt, and even before she reached the bottom step, I had already suggested that she might want to change into some trousers as it was so cold outside. She shook her head, and I could see she would be digging her heels in about this and was clearly very attached to wearing that particular skirt. When she was younger, we might have stood there for twenty minutes while we both tried to persuade each other that we were right. This time I took a different approach.

'We're going on this dog walk,' I said. 'You can wear that skirt if you want, but you will get cold and wet in it. Or you can get changed into trousers and reduce the chances of that happening. But if you decide to go with the skirt, you can't complain about being cold and wet because you now know it was likely to happen.'

She looked unimpressed and told me that she was going to wear the skirt as she thought it was pretty. I shrugged my shoulders and said, 'It's your choice.'

We went on our walk, and it began to rain. The coastal

wind blew, and after a while, even our dog didn't look too pleased to be outside, so we decided to take the shorter route. India did get cold and wet, but when she began complaining about it, I gently reminded her that she had decided to wear the skirt, and this was the consequence. The next day when we took the dog out, she arrived at the top of the stairs in trousers.

As a parent, partner or friend, it can be very easy to tell the people we care about what we think they should do with their lives. It can become a habit for many of us, as we think we're looking out for them, but before we know it, we are commenting on every micro-decision they are facing. This might come from a place of love or protectiveness, but ultimately it will hinder them as we all learn more by making mistakes than by being told what to do. Someone might justify their advice by saying, 'I don't want you to make the same mistakes I did.' But they would have lived a different life in other circumstances, so their experiences won't necessarily apply to other people's lives. This is particularly true with advice from parents on work and money, as they are from an older generation and their examples might come from a very different era. We now live in rapidly changing times, and are often going into uncharted territory. We have to be left to make wrong moves ourselves; we can't just go through life avoiding every hurdle we face, to try to make the journey 'easier'.

Often, the more challenging the journey, the more transformative the growth. Rather than passing on what we've learned, our job is to empower those we care about so that they can make decisions themselves. Our job as parents is not to teach our children a thousand lessons. Our job is to give them the tools to make the wisest decisions for themselves.

Constantly involving yourself in other people's decisions disempowers them by making them believe they cannot make their own choices. All it does is reinforce the idea they are either lacking in essential skills or incapable of rational thinking.

If you are someone who has grown up in an environment where you have always been told what to do, you might find it challenging to start directing your own life. It might be time to make a decision. Do you want to take control of your journey, or do you want others to do it for you? Making your next mistake might be one of the best things you ever do.

Lesson 32: Don't Worry About Tomorrow, Focus on Today

It was the night before Run 4 Nations, my attempt to become the first person in history to run a marathon in all four UK countries within twenty-four hours, and I was in the middle of a minor crisis. Even though I had previously completed several challenges and raised tens of thousands of pounds for charity, I still didn't have a kit sponsor. Usually, with these types of challenges, a sponsor will provide your gear and donate to the charity you are raising money for. I had waited until the last minute, but no company had stepped forward. It felt like everything I had trained for was going unnoticed, and I would be letting the charity down. In the end, I had no other option but to get in my car, feeling completely demoralized, and drive to Sports Direct to buy enough running clothes to allow me to change multiple times while journeying between the four countries.

I think the main reason I didn't have a kit sponsor was because none of the major media outlets had picked up on the story. It was exactly a year after I had run around my patio in lockdown, and I was about to launch myself into one of my biggest challenges with no kit or media coverage. It was a very humbling experience.

Rather than worrying about what would happen the

next day though, I decided to focus on what I could do immediately to improve the circumstances I had found myself in. So, after my trip to Sports Direct, which was luckily still open, I called Megan at the PR agency I was working with. I explained the situation and asked if she could help me prepare a press release. She was the one person I believed could get across the media lines late in the day to promote this, and she ended up doing an exceptional job. The story was picked up by a few outlets, and the donations started pouring in. A few days after completing the run, I checked the fundraising page and was happy to see that we had managed to raise £27,000 for the Samaritans. It would have been so easy to sit there feeling sorry for myself or angry at the situation, but rather than spiral into those emotions I chose to act on what I could control.

When we are faced with the prospect of failure, we might be unable to change our fate completely, but we can at least make a start. As someone with an anxiety disorder, I know how easy it is to fall into a cycle of worrying, but I've learned over the years that thinking too much about tomorrow doesn't ever ease my anxiety, it only exacerbates it. Anxiety often stems from worrying about the future, so when I find myself falling into this trap I try to remind myself of this quote: 'Worried about tomorrow, they forget about today. In the end, they live neither today nor tomorrow.'

What does ease my anxiety is doing something productive, however small, in the here and now – such as cleaning, as it gives me a sense of control. When I feel like my mind is going at a hundred miles an hour about all the things I haven't done, it can feel like nothing will ever be enough and I'll always feel like this, so I've found that it's important to slow things down and have more patience when it comes to my mental health. Am I going to cure or significantly reduce my anxiety today? Probably not, because it's so substantial. So, instead, I ask myself, 'What action can I take today to help with tomorrow?'

Lesson 33: Try Not to Dwell on the Past

My anxiety is exacerbated by worrying about the future, but my previous depression increased when ruminating on the past. I had to remind myself of this recently when a friendship I'd had for a long time came to an end. There were quite a few stages to the implosion of this relationship. It progressively got worse over several months until we ended up not speaking to each other. From my experience of these situations, they usually come down to one of two things: someone's behaviour or money. In this case, it was both, and sadly what was a long-standing friendship is now finished.

When this sort of thing happens, we can waste a lot of energy wondering *why* it happened. I've realized that the answer is because we're all different. Other people will not think and act in the way I do, because they have a distinct set of experiences and values. They won't respond in the way I would want or expect them to, and that's just the reality of life. The most productive route is to accept that and move on, instead of being frustrated by their reaction or the repercussions of their actions. In these cases I genuinely know that I will have to let go of this situation because it will do more damage to me by holding on to it.

I sometimes wonder what my life would be like if I didn't have anxiety or hadn't been depressed. What would be different now? What choices would I have made? It is the same with my undiagnosed ADHD, as I sometimes wonder whether it has held me back. I have always wanted to be an actor, but shied away from pursuing it because I knew it would require memorizing lines and I find it difficult to hold information. If I worked hard, perhaps I would improve my memory, but I would never be on the same level as someone who is naturally gifted in this area. But I have learned that there is no point in dwelling on what could have been. Instead, I have to accept myself for who I am and make the best of what I've got.

The reality is there will always be losses and missed opportunities in life, but what's important is not obsessing about them. We can be upset by what happened today or angered by it, because that's a normal reaction. But eventually, we will have to process that experience or those feelings will remain. If we're still mulling over something years later and haven't a nice word to say, that toxicity will define and envelop us. It will lead us to pushing people away, and we will become isolated.

If we constantly live in the past and dwell on these moments, we will become a victim of them. Being a victim inspires no one. As I talked about in chapter 17 about Tano, people are either drawn to or repelled by the energy we put into the world. No matter what we've been through in life, if we radiate positive energy, we will forever draw people to us.

We also cannot grow as individuals if we're always living in the past. There are so many good things that could come our way, but we cannot free ourselves to recognize, experience or enjoy them if we're not living in the present.

Rather than focusing your energy and animosity on something you've lost, look at what you've gained, which is removing a person or situation from your life that is no longer the right fit for you, or never was in the first place. If they have already caused you worry and trouble, you're better off without them. You no longer have to channel your precious time or resources towards them — they don't get any more of you or your time.

Taking this step to free yourself will open up space in your life to invest your energy into someone worthy of it. This might be someone new, or it could be reconnecting with someone from your past who is aligned with your way of viewing the world — just like my experience in the next chapter.

Lesson 34: Hold On to Those Who You Truly Align With

A good friend of mine is a wedding photographer. When he was in his late teens or early twenties, he had a brief relationship with someone he really liked, but they separated for various reasons. Quite quickly, he found himself in another relationship that lasted ten years. It was clear to me and his other friends that it was not fulfilling him, as his energy dropped and his presence lessened. Eventually he couldn't see any joy in the weddings he photographed, and became pessimistic about marriage, which contradicted what he was trying to achieve with his work. He was trying to showcase and represent the power and unity of love, but couldn't appreciate it himself.

One day we met up, and something big had clearly happened. He had been listening to the speeches at a wedding he was photographing, and something the groom had said had hit him hard. The way the groom had spoken about his bride was so sincere and moving that my friend realized he wasn't in the right relationship. He made the tough decision to talk to his partner about it, and they agreed to separate.

A few weeks later, the girl he'd dated years ago reached out to him. They decided to meet and found that the connection and spark they both remembered still existed. They began a new relationship and moved in together after six months. He joined me on some of my challenges, and one day when we'd been away for a week I asked him if he minded being away from his girlfriend. He replied, 'Every time I leave her is when I am at my saddest.' He had gone from not seeing the value in love at all to feeling it so deeply. If he hadn't made that tough decision to end his long-term relationship, he would never have found the love of his life.

What happened to him reminds me of the quote by the philosopher Albert Schweitzer: 'In everyone's life, at some time, our inner fire goes out. It is then burst into flame by an encounter with another human being. We should all be thankful for those people who rekindle the inner spirit.'

You are likely to have a few people from your past who you still think about, whether former friends or ex-partners. For whatever reason, you drifted apart, then life got in the way, and you realize it's been years since you last spoke to them. The timing might not have been right before if it was a relationship, or you both might have been too busy if it was a friend. It could even be a family member or friend who you still see occasionally but have realized that you don't see them enough.

If there is someone like that who you think would benefit your life and you don't see enough, it might be time to send them a message or make a call. If there is space in your life to put energy into a relationship or friendship, it might be beneficial to rekindle one from your past with someone you already know you're aligned with, or one from your present with someone you don't see enough of. These people are invaluable, and the chance of bringing one of them back into your life and spending more time with them is definitely worth the energy it would take to make a phone call or send a message.

Lesson 35: Restructure Your Norm

Running a marathon every day sounds quite extreme, and even though I have done it I can recognize how crazy it sounds. But as someone who used to hate running, I think it's all a matter of perspective.

The world has become so reliant on technology that so many of us spend the majority of our day sitting down in front of a screen at work, school, or even at home in our spare time. If that is your everyday experience, running a marathon might seem like a vast amount of exercise and probably something you could never achieve. But when you think about it, what is a long distance and what isn't? It's only because there is so much emphasis on the marathon distance being a long way that we see it as something unattainable. If we shift our perspective slightly, what feels impossible can become possible.

If we consider the whole of human history, it's only in the past few decades that we've spent so much time not moving. Our bodies are the product of hundreds of thousands of years of evolution, which enabled us to hunt and gather food, and we would have covered huge distances each day to chase down our food, scavenge or explore. Don't get me wrong, I'm not saying that if you haven't run or exercised for a long time that you could just get up and complete a marathon, because that would be a big shock to your system and potentially cause more harm than good. But I am proof that people can go from never running more than 5k to running 76 consecutive marathons – so, with some training and a bit of motivation, I'm sure you could do it too.

I had to do a lot of training for my first marathon, but it helped me to think of it as getting my body back into the condition it was designed for. I also had to find a way to occupy my ADHD mind, and I quickly realized that the environment I ran in was crucial, and that outdoors in nature with lots to look at was the best place for me to train. Once my body adapted to what I needed it to do each day, I honestly could have continued running for much longer than 76 marathons, because that was my norm. We only think of marathon distances as ridiculously long because we emphasize the length compared to us not doing any exercise. In fact, with some training, most people are capable of completing a marathon. It sounds crazy, but running a marathon every day became my norm; rather than getting up and going to the office at nine and finishing at six, I would wake up, run a marathon from nine until three, rest, get some sleep and do it again the next day. For two and a half months, it was my job.

I know this is extreme, but it just proves how malleable our bodies and minds are – that we are capable of things we never thought possible if we put time into shifting our perception of 'normal'. I don't just mean physically, either. For example, it might be more difficult to set up a business without a degree, but when you think about all the millions of successful companies that have been established in the past thousand years (and are being created right now) by people in similar situations, it doesn't seem so unachievable. It's only in the last few decades that university education has been so accessible, so why should that be a barrier? It didn't stop me!

It's the same thing with diet. Rather than changing everything overnight, it's about making small changes that are more likely to last and reminding ourselves that in a few weeks this will become part of what our body expects, and we'll start looking forward to more nutritious food. I used to know a guy who was heavily addicted to drugs, alcohol, gambling . . . everything you could think of. He got sober and clean, stopped gambling and all his other vices, and started doing ultra-running. He had decided that as he seemed to have an addictive personality, he would switch his focus and do something beneficial that made him feel good. He didn't overtrain, but he did use his addictive personality to help keep himself motivated.

When you focus on the entire task ahead of you, it can be anxiety-inducing. You can become fixated on the end result, whether it's running your first marathon, saving for a mortgage or learning a new language. Of course, that's likely to stress you out, because it can seem enormous when you look at it in its entirety. But if you break it down into what you've got to do that day, it feels far more achievable. This is what it's all about: restructuring your norm, making it a part of your everyday, and gradually shifting your perspective.

Another thing that can make or break you is competition, and we'll talk about that more in the next chapter.

Lesson 36: Being Competitive Can Motivate or Debilitate

My daughter, India, has fallen in love with running too. She has the ability to excel at it, and her eagerness to learn and improve is exciting. Sports day is a big thing for her, and this year she was pipped to the finish by a boy. She came away incredibly frustrated, and when I asked her about this, she responded that she could have done better. I asked her if she had given it everything, and she confirmed she had. I told her that if you come away from anything after giving it your all, the place you finish is irrelevant. All you can do is work on the things you feel could have improved and see if it makes a difference next time. The worst thing to do is focus on the final result and think that if you don't win, the rest doesn't matter. That's nonsense. As I told India, we need to enjoy the process of improving together, and if she doesn't win next year, we can try again if she still wants to.

We are often taught from a young age that we should try to be the best at everything. Of course, in certain settings competition can be important, but it can also detract from the experience. If I'd had to run the 76 Marathons with twenty other runners competing against me, it would have been a completely different experience. Every decision I made would have had a consequence. The smallest detail could have made the difference between winning or losing the race. I would have found myself fixated on energy snacks, pace and timetables. For better or worse, adding an element of competition to anything you are doing significantly increases what is at stake.

I was recently talking to another runner who had set himself a huge running challenge that focused on distances rather than timings. The attention the challenge and his approach to it was getting was playing on his mind, and he was getting nervous about the time it would take him to run. I asked him whether, if he gave himself the option to walk when he needed to, would that take the weight off his shoulders? He replied that it would. One simple option can change everything, and there are solutions for any mental hurdle we create.

We are so used to seeing everything as a competition – comparing our achievements to other people's and putting unnecessary pressure on ourselves. But if we remove the element of competition and say that we are just trying to achieve something for ourselves, then pursuing a goal becomes a process we can enjoy.

We also need to be careful about getting too caught up in a competition with ourselves. I've seen people at the finish line of races in tears because they did not achieve their intended time. That focus on personal bests can affect our mindset. Even setting foot on the start line is an accomplishment in itself, because we need to appreciate the sacrifice and time it took to get to that point. A marathon is a beautiful thing, but it comes with a price.

The experience isn't easy, but the reward of taking part in it can be life-changing.

Learning to love the experience rather than just focusing on the end goal is the key to living a pretty content and fulfilled life – and that's worth more than the validation of reaching the finish line three seconds sooner. Taking the competition element away also makes a goal or challenge more accessible to people, and that's why we didn't include it in the 76 Marathons. We just wanted people to turn up and enjoy running with us.

There's a balance to being competitive, as it can be debilitating and even overwhelm us into inaction. But competition is a great motivator as well. We can use it to spur us on, but we have to be aware of the potential negative effect it can have. It also shouldn't take over the enjoyment of what we are doing. Competition doesn't mean being the fastest, longest or most successful. Competition can also mean striving to do something hard, in which case the completion of the achievement is what signals success.

Lesson 37: Showing Vulnerability Isn't a Weakness – It's a Strength

A moment I will forever remember is when I was running Marathon 39, in Norwich, and a lad in his forties joined me. He was a former soldier raised in a tough home. His father had worked offshore on oil rigs for long stretches of time, which he'd found hard as a child as every time he said goodbye it felt like a lifetime before he would see his dad again. On one occasion he was crying, and his father shouted at him to stop crying as he was the man of the house in his absence and needed to support his mother and sister. From that moment on, he did as he was told and suppressed his emotions. As he went on to become a soldier, he carried this lesson with him. Many years later, when his colleague took his own life, he showed no emotion when he found out. Shocked by his lack of reaction to this painful experience, his partner took him aside and refused to allow it to go on anymore. She would not have him raise their children with this detached mindset. Her words triggered something in him, and at that moment, he broke down. All those years of suppressed emotions came out and this continued for a few days.

He had seen the challenge I was doing and came to connect with me and share his story. He said that he had seen me emotional at several points, which had normalized the way he felt and didn't make him feel weak. He said his relationship with his partner and children was so happy and healthy now. I was so moved by his story, particularly as the Run41Million challenge had played a part in normalizing the emotions he was feeling, but it also made me think: why is this not the same for every man?

Society has taught men that whenever we struggle, we should bottle it up, push down what we feel and keep it to ourselves. But the consequences of that thinking are huge, and are not being dealt with quickly enough. According to government research, the male suicide rate in England is 16.1 per 100,000, compared to a female suicide rate of 5.3. Every man born into this world has emotions, but so few have been taught how to process them. If the narrative around our emotions remains the same, so will this negative cycle.

Marathon 45, in Lichfield, was a poignant run for me. This was the first time the pain I was in became so overbearing it forced me to stop and walk for long periods. I had no idea at the time, but I had a stress fracture in my left foot. Shifting the weight to my right foot put pressure on my right calf, and eventually, it gave in, and the calf tore. Being forced to slow down and spend time on my own gave me more time to be present and process my thoughts. As I worked through the pain, the difficulties of the past couple of years rose to the surface, and I broke down in tears. I could not stop crying. I cried for an entire half marathon.

Touching the door to the cathedral to finish the marathon was a significant moment for me. I was in a vulnerable state, and my pace setter, Chris, came over and sat next to me. A former marine and an incredibly tough man, he put his arm around me and pulled me in tight for a hug. Words weren't needed in that moment, just his acknowledgement of what I was feeling. I didn't want to hear that everything would be 'okay', I just needed to let what I was feeling out of me. There was no judgement from Chris, just empathy, respect and support. It made me feel closer to him, understood and respected, and I was able to face the next day with a stronger mindset.

You can be masculine and still show vulnerability. One doesn't cancel the other out. We currently have a generation of men being raised with an ideology of masculinity that is all about having money, a nice car, living a lavish lifestyle and hooking up with women. But, at least to my mind, these things don't bring you fulfilment or happiness. Young men who have all these things might say that they love their lives, but if you dig down, it's likely that those things are compensation for something lacking on a deeper emotional level. It's a very narrow-minded view of what it means to be a man and I think we owe it to the next generation to give them a fuller picture. One that shows it is normal to have emotions, to cry when you say goodbye to your family or your friend dies. One that enables you to acknowledge that not everything will go your way, but you have the resources to face any tough times head-on.

It is a great privilege of mine that men often feel comfortable reaching out to me about their mental health because of the work I do. Actions, for me, do speak louder than words. I'm not telling someone how to feel or think. Instead, I'm showing them that it's okay to be vulnerable. It has taken me six years to get to this point of understanding myself, and to see that change having an impact on others too. It has always been my aim to create a space that's safe and without judgement. There is no right or wrong. I just present my approach, and if you connect with that, then great. If you don't or aren't ready to, that's equally fine. I'll still be here when you're ready.

If we allow our emotions to surface when they need to, they can be processed and allowed to pass. They aren't given the chance to gather inside us and pull us down into a place we might struggle to recover from. It can be painful to meet them head-on, especially when they have been pushed down for so long, but that is why showing vulnerability isn't a weakness – it's a strength.

Lesson 38: Create a Space That Calms You

I have learned that living in London isn't the ideal place for my mental well-being. Outside my front door is a hectic city running at an incredibly fast pace that I find overstimulating. I used to get burned out very quickly just from a day getting to work and back; and when you add in looking after a child, picking them up from school, and juggling everything when they are ill or don't sleep well, it can take its toll and, if I'm not careful, impact my mental health. One way that I have learned to combat this is by creating a space at home that relaxes me, and I had to make some adjustments to it to try to make it as beneficial as possible.

I have a tiny patio and a relatively small space that I call home, but I've tried to enhance this as best I can. For me, it's all about creating connections and memories inside my home. I connect with the outdoors by having indoor plants. On my patio, I have three olive trees that remind me of the places abroad such as Italy that I have visited and fallen in love with. I also have plants that were chosen because their scent aids mental well-being. At the end of the John O'Groats to Land's End challenge, I visited the Eden Project with my family. In the Mediterranean section was a particular type of lavender from Greece that India was obsessed with. I bought some and planted it in my garden, to remind me of that special day and of India's reaction to finding a plant that she loved.

I find bright colours stressful, and they make my brain jumpy, so I try to use neutral tones that calm my mind and remind me of the ocean. It's not about trying to kid myself that I'm by the ocean; it's about feeling connected to it. I grew up by the coast, and one of my favourite things in the world is the sea. I couldn't be happier or more present than when I'm in water, and most of my fondest memories are either in the sea or beside it. Everyone has a noise that soothes them, and for me, it is the sound of the waves outside my bedroom window.

I also find it really grounding and relaxing to have photos around me, so that when I see them it prompts happy memories, leaving less space for anxious thoughts. In the hallway of my apartment, there is a wall of framed photos of important times in my life that make me feel good. When I wake up in the morning and open my bedroom door, they are the first thing I see and this is how I start my day. You don't have to change everything in your home; it doesn't take much to change an oppressive environment into a sanctuary. It's just about finding simple ways to trigger happy memories.

This also really helps me when I'm travelling, particularly if I'm on a lengthy challenge. I will take small reminders with me to help create a temporary home. During the 76 Marathons, there was always a framed picture of me and India and one of her teddies sat at the end of my bed. By the halfway mark, our camper van began to feel like home, and I was happier sleeping there than on the occasions we were offered a hotel for the night. The reminder of India made it feel like home. It was a tiny space filled with three or four men, but even in those cramped conditions, it became a place of peace. It was somewhere we felt settled and could try to recover from what we had been through that day.

That's what a home is for me, whether temporary or permanent. It is somewhere that makes me feel secure, so my mind can relax for a few hours and recover.

Lesson 39: Test Your Limits, but Know Your Limitations

I've been doing challenges for around six years and can already see the changes happening. The numbers are growing. People clearly want to test themselves, which is exciting and encouraging. The caveat to this is that it seems that people feel they need to go bigger in order to be seen or heard. This is when it can start to cross into unhealthy territory, and the risk can outweigh the reward.

I've thought about this often and wondered how we know when we're going too far. My opinion is that as soon as I am risking my life or going to cause irreversible damage to my body, then it's not worth it. I don't want to cause a long-term impact on my quality of life or place a huge burden on my family who will have to care for me. Nothing we set ourselves to achieve is worth our lives, and undervaluing our lives that easily doesn't make sense to me. But it seems that people are getting closer to that boundary.

My daughter plays a large part in the view that I take because of my responsibility towards her, both to be there as a father and to ensure that she isn't impacted by my decisions. She gives me enormous purpose and is a clear reminder of how precious life is. Being mindful of her doesn't mean I won't push myself and test my limits, however. The fact I ran more than thirty marathons with a stress fracture and torn calf shows the lengths I'm willing to go to, but I wouldn't put my life at risk, even to raise money for charity. I'm also fortunate to be surrounded by qualified professionals who protect me by keeping an eye on my limits.

Others might think differently, and that's their choice, but I don't believe we should feel obliged to push ourselves beyond what is reasonably safe. At some point, taken to its extremes, it becomes a gladiatorial contest of whether someone will survive or not. We shouldn't feel pressured to risk our lives to promote awareness of a cause or raise money for charity. I also don't think charities would want us to do this for them. Therefore, we need to consider the point where it tips over from being productive to potentially destructive.

I see this behaviour in the Ultimate Fighting Championships (UFC), where seven fighters have died in the ring since 2019. Some of the fighters say in interviews that they are willing to die in that octagon, and I think they really mean it. It makes me wonder how much they have to live for if they are willing to throw their lives away for the chance of victory.

My opinion is that there must be a balance between inspiring people to go above and beyond and knowing when to stop. It's about considering the cost and impact that something going wrong will have on those around you. Although it's incredibly valuable to pursue your interests and ambitions, you also need to be mindful of the people around you and try to find a balance so they aren't hurt by your decisions. If you're living a regimented life that revolves around strict training, or long hours and no joy or connection with other people, I think something might be missing.

Obviously, not everyone reading this book will find themselves in the position of testing themselves in an extreme, or potentially dangerous, challenge. However, we can do just as much damage to ourselves and our longevity in small, incremental steps when we work long days in stressful jobs or sit down all day, or when we stretch ourselves too thin by juggling looking after children and endless other demands on our time. There is only so much we can change when these roles and expectations are placed on us, but we have to be aware of the damage they can do to our health and our relationships, and to take a break when we can.

No matter what challenge we want to achieve, we all need to test our limits. If we don't push ourselves, we will never know how far we can go. But we also need a clear idea of what and where our limitations are and draw lines for ourselves early on that we won't cross. We should ringfence what is safe and responsible in terms of all our competing needs, and take a break when necessary. The last thing we want is to become fixated on an outcome and throw everything else aside, to the detriment of ourselves or those close to us. While we all need to push ourselves, it's just as important to learn when to stop.

Lesson 40: It's Not About the Size of the Challenge, It's the Connection

It wasn't until I started the 76 Marathons that I truly cracked what would inspire more of the general public to join in, get behind what I was doing and, ultimately, help me raise more money. The challenge was potentially accessible to them as it was in every city in the United Kingdom, and there were daily updates on what we were doing. We could have run a marathon in every city in the world, but without people knowing about it and believing in it, it would have been missing one vital ingredient – connection.

This experience taught me that if you want people to pay attention to what you're doing, then you have to build a connection with them. They have to understand the reasoning behind your mission, and it must produce an emotional response that might even inspire them to take action.

This applies to whatever you are trying to achieve, if it involves the need for people to know about it. If you're setting up a new business and want people to buy your services or product, there has to be a connection with the public, or they will buy from someone else. If you want to raise awareness of an unjust law and begin a campaign around it, the public need to be aware of what you are doing, as you are more likely to make a change if you have public opinion supporting you. If you want to raise money and awareness for a charity by completing a challenge, that connection has to be in place, or people won't be moved to take action and donate.

If you go into something that needs people's eyes on it, but you don't have the necessary social media or net-working skills to create this, or the ability to connect with people through your message, it is unlikely to get the attention it deserves. On a personal level, you will still gain a lot from it, which is hugely valuable and not to be dismissed. But if the desired outcome is to raise money for charity or encourage awareness of a cause or business, people need to hear about what you're trying to do and get behind it, which all comes down to con-nection. You will need to excel at that element, as well as all the things involved in what you're trying to achieve.

It took me a long time, and a lot of trial and error, to learn this, but it's now fundamental to my work.

The first part of creating a connection is awareness. People have to know about what you're doing if you're going to have a chance of them caring about it. You can have the best business or challenge in the world, but if no one knows about it, they can't get behind it. This means you have to talk about it, and share it with as many people as you can. Nirmal Purja climbed the fourteen 'Death Zone' peaks in under seven months in 2019, but was only truly recognized for his achievement two years later when a Netflix documentary about it was released.

Recently, Kristin Harila has now beaten that record with the Nepalese mountaineer Tenjen Sherpa, by climbing those same fourteen peaks in just three months.

Once you have awareness, there can be a connection. The narrative behind what you are doing will normally beat the extremeness of it, hands down.

The next part is frequency, and creating continued awareness. In my early challenges, I tried weekly documentaries on YouTube. They looked great and were beautifully shot and engaging, but the gap between them was too long. There wasn't that real-time engagement; there have to be regular updates to keep people invested in what you're doing on a daily basis. I found that a weekly eight-minute documentary was too much, too late. There's so much else going on in the world that we can all easily move on to the next thing if we have to wait days between updates. Streaming platforms will release a whole or half a season at a time now because of this. We need continuous investment.

The third part is showing the reality of the situation you find yourself in. It can't all be portrayed as either constant achievements or continuous setbacks, because that's not how these things work. There are highs and lows, and people need to see the full range of your experiences. It's normal for people to make judgements when they first become aware of you, but if these assumptions aren't true, you will need to correct them by showing what you're really going through.

There has to be authenticity in what you do. People want

to see the reality of what you experience. I know that when people look at me and become aware of my history, they think I'll be tackling these challenges in comfort and luxury to ease myself through them. In reality, I go feral on challenges, and there was even an intervention on one because I smelled so bad. I don't like to feel groomed during these challenges because the reality is you're waking up to torrential rain that you have to spend the day in. What you don't want to do is be in a fancy hotel where you're waking up to a hot shower and a full English, because that actually makes the adjustment to the day you're facing much harder. I'm in my element when I'm half-wild, barefoot, and waking up in a remote area where I can step outside into a natural landscape. People tell me they don't understand how I've done some of my challenges. What they don't realize is that I'm happiest in this kind of environment. All it takes is a bit of greenery and any type of water, and I'm filled with so much joy. Comfort and luxury are rarely my priorities outside of challenges, and certainly never my priority when I'm in the middle of them.

If you want to achieve something just for yourself, then that is a great ambition to have and hugely beneficial. You don't need to publicize what you're doing if you don't want to. But if what you're doing requires public support because you're raising money for charity, championing a cause or starting up a business, then you do need to think about how to build that connection. Because to gain people's support, you need to give them a reason that really connects.

Lesson 41: We Don't Need to Tell Everyone Everything

One of my friends is a really talented artist who was making waves in the art world. She was gaining attention, and her career was beginning to take off. On the advice of someone at her gallery, she contacted a PR company who said they could get her interviews in media outlets or on podcasts. But there was a catch – she was advised to talk about her experiences as a recovering addict. When she told me about this, it was clear she was torn. She knew that revealing this type of story about herself would help people connect with her, but she also didn't feel comfortable talking about it on a public platform. It seemed like a big opportunity, but I reminded her that she was already being recognized for her art without this press. I asked her, 'What do you want to be known for? Do you want to share that as part of your story, or for your work to be recognized regardless of that?' She wanted the latter.

She decided not to go down that path and to instead build her credibility in the art world, make a real success of what she was doing and widen her audience that way. In the future, it would be her choice whether she revealed this information about herself. If she did decide to communicate that message later on, with an even larger audience the impact would be even greater.

Although I believe we should all be more accepting of and open about our struggles, I am wary of how we talk about them. I've struggled with my mental health, but I don't make that my sole identity – it's just a part of my story. When I approach a challenge, I'm raising money for charity, which is often linked to mental health awareness, prevention or assistance. My reasoning behind this is that I never want the topic to feel like a weight on someone's shoulders. Showcasing the Why that has inspired my challenges is key, so people can understand the passion behind the cause.

The behaviour social media can produce is genuinely concerning. Its use can provoke extreme behaviour to satisfy algorithms and achieve reach and engagement. But we have a choice about how we create content and engage with other users.

Whatever it is that you are trying to achieve, if you do decide to talk about it in a public way, you get to control the narrative. What we choose to share about ourselves is our decision to make, and we shouldn't feel pressured to reveal more than we're comfortable with. We don't have to tell everyone everything.

Lesson 42: Hold On to the People You Care About

I was at a wedding recently and was really pleased to bump into a friend there who I hadn't spoken to in years. I went over and gave her a big hug, and then we proceeded to catch up on each other's lives and all the major events that had taken place. When I mentioned that it was ridiculous that we hadn't even messaged each other in years, she didn't seem as surprised as I was about the length of time it had been. It was then that she told me that she had decided to stop texting me three years ago to see if I ever made the effort to contact her. I never did. I had disconnected from that friendship without even realizing it.

This really bothered me, because I hadn't intentionally not put the effort in, but the outcome was the same. It was the classic story of 'life just got in the way'. Even though contacting her wasn't at the top of my list, she was often in my thoughts, but I hadn't done anything about it.

I really respected the way my friend approached the situation. There was no drama or accusations. Anyone at the wedding who saw us talking would have just thought we were two old friends having a pleasant conversation. She told me what had happened from her perspective in a straightforward, non-confrontational way. I was unaware of the decision she had made three years ago, but she didn't expect me to have any knowledge of it; she had just consciously decided to take a step back and wait for me to reach out to her, and I hadn't. How she articulated herself helped me learn something from what she was saying rather than making me feel as if I had to defend myself and it snowballing into an argument. She gave me time to process what she had said and waited patiently for my response, which was to apologize. Because she took this approach, a friendship was saved and will continue for many years.

This revelation gave me a chance to reflect on what I'd done and make amends, not just with her but with many people. The following week I made a list of people I truly valued in my life and dropped them a message. It didn't take very long, but it let them know they were in my thoughts.

In the case of my friend at the wedding, she hadn't heard from me because I had been through a pretty turbulent time in my life after separating from the mother of my child. But the lack of contact was still my fault, and I fully accepted it. Luckily there was enough understanding, patience and recognition of how best to communicate with the other person that we could have that difficult conversation. At the time I hadn't been reaching out, I was just trying to get through each day. Many people close to me were neglected, which I'm deeply sorry for. The truest friends stuck around or would eventually understand the reasons behind my absence. Those who left were not meant to be. Although those moments in life are challenging to go through, the friends who are invested in you will stand by you.

Our time is limited, and we become more aware of this as we get older. Regrets come from a lack of something. It might be an unrealized dream or losing a connection we once had. Having people around us who bring something positive to our life enriches the quality of it, and we should try to keep them around us rather than letting them drift away. It's important to try to prioritize the friendships that are important to us.

The individuals we surround ourselves with will influence our mindset. Therefore, we should actively choose them rather than allowing circumstances to select them for us.

Lesson 43: You Need at Least One Person in Your Life Who Will Tell You the Hard Truth

My mum is my rock. Whenever I have a problem or am unsure what to do, I turn to her for advice. I don't do this because she tells me what I want to hear. I do this because she's level-headed, and nine times out of ten will tell me what I don't want to hear.

Being confronted with the hard truth about a situation can be incredibly annoying. I've been there many times, when I just wanted confirmation that I was right or that what I achieved was great and I can move on to the next thing. The last thing I want to hear is that I have to revisit something or start again. But from my experience, after I've had a chance to let it sink in, I'll accept what my mum is saying. This is because, annoying as it might be, she's usually right.

Standing up and telling someone the hard truth takes strength, which I admire about my mum. She'd have an easier life if she didn't do this for me, but she loves me enough to tell me the truth.

I appreciate everyone in my life who cares enough about me to tell me their honest opinion. Hearing what they have to say can also be humbling, and we all need

a bit of humility at times, or we can easily lose ourselves. Whenever I've done documentaries or made
something that is important to me, I always fill the
room with people who will tell me the truth. I've got
no interest in people telling me that a documentary is
the best thing they've ever seen when it isn't. That
doesn't help the outcome that I'm trying to achieve.
Ultimately, I need honesty if I want to be the best version of myself and create something that will inspire
others. I want to know whether something passes the
standards I set for myself, and if it doesn't, I want to
know how we can make it better.

True friends should want the best for us, and this means
telling us the truth or where we can improve when necessary. This isn't the same as being hyper-critical, as that
often comes from either a projection about what they are
feeling within themselves or a place of envy. Anyone can
be critical and find something negative to say – criticizing
things is surprisingly easy to do. But that isn't productive,
and can undermine a person's confidence and eventually tear them down. Even if it's done with the best
intentions, if you constantly critique someone, they'll
eventually switch off from you and not listen to anything you say, and you'll lose the chance you had to help
them. Criticism should be balanced against highlighting
what someone has done well, so that they can see that
you are also acknowledging their achievements.

How people communicate their feedback is also
important. We can have so much knowledge that we

want to share, but if we don't know *how* to convey it so that it will be absorbed, then there is little point in us raising it. When you want to share something with someone, you should know them well enough to understand the nuances of what they respond well to. You might call them instead of sending a message, or try to make it funny. Making more positive points than negative ones might be the best way to make it land. It's all about finding the best method to deliver the truth so that it reaches the person who needs to hear it.

Lesson 44: Your Thoughts Don't Define You

Although I now love running long distances, this amount of time alone gives you a lot of thinking time – so much so that there is the chance of being overrun by your thoughts. They pop in and out uninvited, and your brain can take you to some of the strangest places. I have never been able to control my thoughts and go into a zen-like trance while running. Instead, my brain bounces around, and it feels like I consider every possibility under the sun. My mind can take me to some pretty dark places, and I've learned to just let it happen and ride it out.

Marathon 42, in Peterborough, was a classic example of this – I set out feeling tired that day and had a bleak mindset. It was midway through the challenge, but it felt like the end was still a long way off, as another thirty-four marathons stretched out in front of me. I'd passed the elation of the halfway mark, which was a huge boost, but that was a few marathons before, and now it felt like I was climbing another steep hill.

Another reason for my negative outlook was, strangely, because I had spent the previous evening with my family. That should have been a positive thing, and it was at the time, but I felt the repercussions the next day. Spending time with my family had shifted my focus away from the challenge, and triggered emotions I had been working so hard to suppress. Although seeing them had brought pure joy, it also weakened me as I was distracted from what I needed to achieve. When I am in the depths of these challenges, the only way I can face them is by closing myself off from home comforts and getting completely in the zone without the distractions of normal life. Consequently, when I woke up the morning after seeing them, my energy was low, which sparked negative thoughts about the route we were taking being testing.

Luckily I had learned from past bouts of anxiety not to panic when my brain runs away with itself like that. We all have thoughts that take us by surprise, such as imagining worst-case scenarios or thinking horrible things about ourselves. This doesn't mean they're true or the events we've imagined will happen. It's just our minds throwing random thoughts out at us that we have to try not to dwell on. This is easier said than done, but it helps me if I try not to get panicked about my thoughts or wonder what they say about me. They're just thoughts. They don't mean that I believe that or that it will happen.

During Marathon 42, I turned those spiralling thoughts into rage and said to my brain that if it thought it could go crazy, I'd show it crazy. I was willing to ride out this phase for as long as it needed. By the end of the day, I was exhausted by what was going on in my head, but then I spotted someone special waiting for me. A family friend had very sadly lost her child to suicide and was waiting patiently for me at the finish line. I went over and gave her the biggest hug I could, as I wanted her to know how grateful I was that she had come to support me. In that moment the Why behind the challenge really hit home. We wanted to raise money and awareness of the work the Samaritans do for people struggling with their mental health, and every few pounds we raised meant another call to their helpline could be answered. All the emotions of the day came crashing in on me, and I told her I needed a minute. I turned around, took some deep breaths, and tried to set aside what was going on in my mind as I thought about the enormity of her situation and what she was living with. That moment reminded me why I had chosen to be there. I was fortunate that I could manage the mental and physical pain that I was going through, but the loss of her son was something she would live with for the rest of her life. This challenge was about honouring her son alongside so many others lost to suicide, and hopefully preventing others from reaching that point. That day was one of the most testing during the challenge, but also one of the most impactful.

Never forget that your thoughts don't define who you are – your actions do. I've learned over the years that if my thoughts try to weaken me, I can counteract them with actions that make me feel stronger.

Lesson 45: Life is an Opportunity

It was early in the morning when Tano called to say he'd had another idea – and in typical Tano fashion, it was something extraordinary. He'd been thinking about the Make-A-Wish Foundation and what they do for children who have been diagnosed with critical conditions. He's a pretty impulsive guy, so he had called the charity and asked them how much money they needed to fulfil wishes for three of these children. They informed him it would be £7,000, and on the spur of the moment, he decided to raise the full amount the same day. Tano's actions define him as a person.

How do you raise £7,000 for charity in one day without any preparation, planning, training or announcements? If there is one man naive enough to start it and stubborn enough to finish it, it's Tano. A month before our call, he had jumped on a bike in his gym to see how his legs would respond to it. With a few cycles under his belt, he now decided that this would be his way to raise the £7,000. He had only cycled a few kilometres in each short session since the accident that damaged his spine, but despite this, he wanted to cycle for as long as it took to raise the money. He had gone from realizing that he could cycle again to deciding to cycle until he raised

£7,000, in a matter of weeks. Because of his injuries, there would almost certainly be physical repercussions for him as well.

So, Tano went to the gym he owns, set up an online donation page and announced that he was going to cycle for as long as it took to raise £7,000 on social media. He then began to pedal. The donations slowly rolled in, but his back became increasingly painful. Despite the discomfort Tano was in, he carried on. He pushed on for several hours, and thankfully momentum built online. The word got out about what he was doing and he managed to raise the full amount in just over eleven hours. When that final donation landed, he got off the bike, his back went into a spasm, and he had to lie down. He was an exhausted but very happy man. He has a mindset I admire and a determination I rarely see.

After Tano's motorbike accident, I had needed to ensure he had something to focus on. I have a very supportive and engaged social media following. So, I suggested to Tano that he document his recovery on his social media accounts to keep him accountable and help people see that their approach to life can affect the outcome. Tano didn't see his accident as a limitation and instead viewed it as the start of something new. His view was that we can't control what's been done, but we can control what comes from it. This inspired so many people, and he gained a very invested following overnight. He even went above and beyond the prediction for his recovery, and learned to walk again. Years after taking his first steps post-accident and no longer needing a wheelchair, he feels a huge amount of gratitude. He's committed his life to giving back in ways both big and small, from riding for eleven hours to raise money for charity to paying for the person behind him at a cafe without them knowing. It's not for a reaction or thanks. He just wants to spread a little joy.

Tano sees his accident and the resulting injuries as something that gave him a deep appreciation for life. Like the rest of us, he hadn't really considered how brief life could be before his injuries; he had been young and wrapped up in the daily distractions of living. But his accident allowed him to appreciate the preciousness of life in a way many never will. Being in hospital for so long meant he met people from all walks of life and was exposed to the realities of different people's existences. When he eventually left hospital, he no longer saw his injuries as a limitation. Instead, he recognized that he had been given a second chance and saw that as an opportunity to help others. He had seen how reliant on others we can become when we are ill or injured, and this inspired him to support those who need it whenever he could.

Tano had gained an extraordinary gift of compassion and appreciation for life from being in a life-threatening accident, but we can learn a lot regardless of our own experiences by slowing down and taking time to consider how fleeting life is. When we take a step back and think of the hundreds of thousands of years humans have been on this planet, our own time on earth becomes equivalent to a grain of sand. We don't have to wait until our life is almost taken from us to appreciate what we have. We all have the opportunity of today, so don't wait until tomorrow.

Lesson 46: Tomorrow is Not Promised

Whenever other runners joined us for the 76 Marathons, we would always try to run together. People naturally run at different paces, but I encouraged everyone to avoid seeing what we were doing as a competition and embrace the communal side. On one particular marathon, a few new people joined us, and we all set off at a steady pace. After around 5 kilometres, someone ran to the front and told me a woman was running quite far behind us. My stance is that if someone has come to join me to run, we do it together. So, I dropped right back and found her, and we began to chat. Yes, she was running quite slowly, but she was also running steadily and didn't look tired or overexerted.

I asked her if she was okay, and she told me that she was absolutely fine but could only run slowly as she had to keep her heart rate down. I asked her why, and she explained that she'd had heart surgery a month ago. This floored me, and I asked if she should be running at all. Her doctors had advised her not to run, she said, but had told her that if she did, she should ensure her heart rate stayed below a certain rate. As we gently jogged side by side, she began to tell me more of her story and why she had wanted to run with us that day.

She had recently been diagnosed with a heart condition that her younger brother had passed away from at the age of three. She had always loved running, so rather than letting this hold her back, she refused to live in fear. Her stance was that having lost someone she loved to this condition she wanted to live her life to the fullest. Although it was a risk to her health, her family and friends admired and respected her for what she was doing. They knew that, ultimately, she was fulfilled, content and happy. She was wary of how much she exerted herself and would never push herself too far, so had decided to keep running even after her surgery. That day, she ended up running with us for 20 kilometres. Then, with a smile and a wave, she dropped out because she knew she had done enough.

Her whole attitude was 'Don't wait for tomorrow, as tomorrow is not promised', which I found inspiring. She had been diagnosed with the condition that had already tragically taken her younger brother's life, but she wasn't going to let the same condition stop her from doing the things she loved. If she was just waiting for her heart condition to flare up, then she might not have lived at all. That was a bold decision to make, and one we all have to think about. Do we live a full life today with no expectancy of a tomorrow? Or do we live an unfulfilled life today while hoping for a better tomorrow? I took inspiration from this woman's approach to life because she chose to be fulfilled rather than living her life in fear.

Tomorrow is not promised. We can never be sure that

it will come, so if we have a good idea of what we want to do (which is often half the battle), we need to get on and do it. Because if we don't, we'll end up regretting it.

Understanding there is no guarantee on how many days I will get always encourages me to take action today. Because I want to *live* rather than just exist.

Lesson 47: Give More to the World Than You Take

A life coach I occasionally see once gave me some poignant advice, which turned out to be a very valuable lesson. She told me that when we do something in life, we should do it because we want to, not because we expect something in return. I like to think of this as we should try to give more to the world than we take from it, and we should also never expect that we are owed anything. If we are happy to do something because we want to do it, we don't ever consider whether we should get something in return – we don't regret or begrudge the action we took.

You can get into real philosophical knots if you consider whether giving to charity or raising money for charitable causes is truly selfless. This is because there is always something you receive in return – it makes you feel fulfilled. You are able to support someone in need, which makes you feel good. It's the same feeling as when I mentor people who come to me with their ideas and plans for the future. I don't get paid for it, but I do get a sense of fulfilment from seeing their growth and witnessing their success. In my case, nothing makes me more fulfilled than helping others feel that same level of fulfilment. So, yes, I get a benefit from it, but I figure that, because I don't expect anything in return – not even that sense of fulfilment – it still qualifies as an intentionally selfless act.

We have to take that first step, though, of taking action and realizing that we contribute to the change we want. I would be a wealthy man if I had a pound for every time someone said to me, 'I tell you what, I don't know what's going to happen to the world when David Attenborough dies.' They're clearly concerned about the environment and value Attenborough's work so much they think it will be almost game over when he passes. The man is in his nineties, and some people saying this to me are in their twenties. What is stopping them from stepping forward and joining that cause to work on supporting the environment in any way they can? Obviously we can't all become environmental presenters, but there are actions we can take such as supporting environmental charities with donations or volunteering, or helping to clean up our local areas. Attenborough cares so much about the environment, but he wants the rest of us to as well. He wouldn't want us to believe we are all doomed once he's gone. No one can ever replace him, but I bet he'd be proud knowing his passion and work inspired someone to try.

This is the thing about giving. It doesn't have to be raising money for charity or making donations. It could be the gift of time spent volunteering or helping others out. Giving comes in many forms, and all of them are valuable. The simple question we all need to ask ourselves is whether we give more than we receive. If the scales are tipping more towards the taking side, then perhaps this needs to be adjusted – not just for the benefit of others but for our own fulfilment as well.

Lesson 48: Make the Most of the Hand You've Been Dealt

At the end of 2019, I had the opportunity of interviewing someone for my podcast who I had first come across on the Netflix documentary *Roll with Me: A Journey across America*. At the time, I was still doing challenges in a wheelchair, so it felt pretty poignant when I was sitting on my sofa one night and a documentary about a man who used a wheelchair appeared on my Netflix suggested list. Documentaries are one of my favourite things to watch, so I got stuck in straight away. A couple of hours later, I was in tears and knew I had to speak with the man who starred in it, Gabriel Cordell. The documentary had really touched me, and I wanted to learn more about him.

When Gabriel was twenty-two years old, he was paralysed from the chest down in a car accident on the way to his first acting audition. After four months in hospital, he was discharged and decided to continue to try to work as an actor even though he was paraplegic. Despite the odds being stacked against him, Gabriel secured some roles. Twenty years passed, and at forty-two, he found a different way to live a fulfilled life. In 2013, he became the first person to cross the United States in a conventional wheelchair rather than a high-tech racing wheelchair. He did this in ninety-nine days, and the 3,100-mile journey took him from California across to New York State. The documentary I had watched followed this journey.

What I found so inspirational about Gabriel's story was that he always did the best he could with what he had. He didn't have a professional team with him, and there was no sponsorship. Instead, he cobbled together a group of misfits with the time and willingness to travel across the country to support him. There were no luxuries on their journey, and they slept in a camper van and ate basic food, but what they did have was pure determination. There was no training involved or a professional team backing him, but he still managed to complete what he had set out to do. Gabriel's approach was that he recognized that he was unbelievably unprepared for this challenge, and the only thing he had on his side was the adversity he had faced and the resilience that created in him. He used that as fuel and continued to push on no matter what.

Gabriel's approach greatly impacted how I viewed my challenges and made me realize that anything is possible, even if you don't have all the pieces in place. At the time, I was preparing to travel by wheelchair from John O'Groats to Land's End, and the only wheelchair I could find had been built and fitted for someone else. I was worried about whether it would impact my ability to complete the challenge. But Gabriel had never had a kit sponsor, a racing wheelchair or a full team of experts, and that hadn't stopped him. He'd travelled across the whole of the United States wearing gardening gloves. This attitude made me take a less rigid view of what was required when approaching my own work. Sometimes people come into your life at precisely the right time, and it isn't something you can ignore. I felt that way about Gabriel – it was as though he was speaking directly to me in that documentary. Without knowing it, he played a massive part in my success in the challenges that followed.

When we face adversity, we can choose how we react to it. Unfortunately, too often, people become victims of their adversity. It can be incredibly hard to push forwards if you don't have the support emotionally or financially; it can be so easy to lose hope and feel isolated. But the most crucial thing in how we deal with adversity is that we accept what has happened and try to make the most of it. Whether it's a physical injury, a setback at work or a relationship coming to an end, trying to fight against what has happened will only lead to more pain. As I've said before, when Tano walks into a room on crutches, he radiates positive energy and doesn't define himself by his disability, so others don't either. He accepted the hand he was dealt six years ago in the accident that damaged his spine, and knows he will never walk in the same way again. But he has also made the most of it, just as Gabriel Cordell did, and both of them are my inspirations.

Lesson 49: Find Time to Connect with the Earth

Most days, many people, including myself, wake up to four walls and a hard floor. We put on shoes, which protect our feet but also disconnect us from the ground. Travelling to work can take us onto fume-filled roads, deep underground, or packed into buses or trams with a hundred others. We might go into an office with bright artificial lighting, and for many people, it's not even a job they enjoy. There might be the chance to glimpse the sky during our lunch break. But we don't look up because we're looking down at our phones, which are always nearby with their bright screens and flickering images as we watch someone else's reality to forget about our own.

It's so easy to feel disconnected from the natural world now, which can unsettle our unconscious minds. The outside world was our home for tens of thousands of years; it's what our bodies and minds still need because we are designed to live in that environment.

As soon as I return to the countryside, I take my shoes and socks off and stay that way for most of the time I'm there. There is nothing quite like walking on grass or sand with nothing between you and the ground. It centres you and makes you feel connected to a larger reality and purpose than your own. You feel part of something bigger, and it, quite literally, grounds you in the present moment.

I always know I have been away from the countryside for too long when it hurts to walk barefoot because the skin on my feet has softened. But after a while, the skin hardens, and I can walk quite comfortably over any surface. I will even go to the pub and meet my friends without shoes on, and no one judges me because they all understand my reasoning and just let me get on with it. Some of them go barefoot too.

Back in the city, I couldn't do this because whenever you do something considered extreme in an urban area, even if it is very normal in another environment, it looks like you are looking for attention. I'd rather wear shoes than let anybody think that what I'm doing is a stunt or a desperate bid for a few eyes on me.

I think it's a big problem in society that we are losing our ability to connect to or have an awareness of the people around us. We lose touch with what we have in common with people who live differently to us, which can make us hostile to one another. What connects us is the ground we walk on and the planet we live on. If we all had more appreciation for and felt more connected to the natural world in our everyday lives, I think we would have more in common with everyone around us and feel more united. Whether it's looking up at the sky and taking a moment to appreciate the moon that millions of others are looking at too, watching the waves that connect us to places thousands of miles away, or just listening to the sounds of the birds that don't recognize borders or boundaries – there are endless ways that we can find peace, beauty and connection in the natural world that surrounds us.

I'm not delusional. I know that for many people the idea of taking their shoes off and walking barefoot might sound quite bizarre or be the last thing they want to do. I've got friends in London who can't think of anything worse than going to the countryside, and they'd raise an eyebrow at the idea of walking barefoot. They live in the fast lane and feel anything below that pace is boring. But I do believe that slowing down and connecting with the earth can be learned if you allow yourself to. Yes, I grew up in the countryside, so it's easier for me, but look at the flip side. I'm a country boy who grew up by the sea, but I've learned how to live in a city and enjoy many aspects of it. I'm making the best of it, and it shows that everyone has the ability to change and learn to appreciate something new.

Lesson 50: Don't be Afraid to Leave the Comfort of What You Know

Around five years ago, my friend's father had just been diagnosed with cancer, and the medication he needed to treat it was astronomically expensive. Wanting to support my friend and her family, I signed up for a white-collar boxing match without much thought of what it would actually involve. It was an easy decision to make, but as the days ticked along, I realized that I had no idea how to box or who my opponent would be. Even though I'd gone into it with the best intentions, I questioned whether I had made a silly decision as I had no boxing experience and little time to prepare for something with a potentially bleak outcome. Visions of me being floored in the first round danced through my mind as my uneasiness grew.

Regardless of what was going through my mind, there was no way I would ever pull out. The Why was bigger than me. What I would face was nothing compared to what my friend and her father were going through. It was natural to feel anxious, but I used that as motivation to train and help my preparation for the fight.

The first big decision I made was not to join the organized group boxing sessions with the other fighters, as I didn't like the idea of my potential competitor learning about my strengths and weaknesses. On the flip side, I knew this meant that I would equally not know about theirs. I would just be banking on my hard work leading up to the fight to prepare me to face my competitor. A few days later, I started my first training session with my new boxing coach, Gary Logan. He was a former professional boxer and a tough coach with an infectious passion for the sport.

I was going through a rough patch at the time following a particularly bad break-up. It had left me feeling incredibly vulnerable and pretty emasculated. Using my anger at the situation in a productive manner was the only way I could cope with it. Meeting Gary was a huge turning point in that chapter of my life.

Going into my training with Gary, I expected to face a series of physical tests. But he began our first session by telling me a story that set the tone from that moment on. When Gary was a kid, he'd had to start at a new school. An older child had decided to make an example of the new boy and ordered Gary to meet him for a fight at the end of the day. This older kid quickly started to throw punches, and Gary ducked and dived and avoided them all – not a single one landed. As this continued, Gary's opponent's confidence began to drop as he realized he had underestimated Gary. This new boy was a complete unknown. If he had done his research first, he might have discovered that Gary came from a boxing family and had been training since he could walk. Gary told me there was a defining moment in the fight where he saw pure fear in the older boy's eyes because he had finally realized that if Gary was skilled enough to duck every punch, what would it be like when he finally threw one? With that realization, the other kid dropped his fists to his sides and walked away. Gary had won a fight without throwing a single punch.

How Gary introduced boxing to me was a testament to his character and his approach of needing the skill to beat an opponent but the restraint of knowing when to use it. Over the following weeks, I learned the same mental discipline from him that I subsequently channelled into so many areas of my life. When you go into a boxing ring, you don't go in filled with rage and aggression. You go in with a clear head and a tactical approach. This was a life-changing skill that I still use to this day. When I find myself in a vulnerable or frustrating situation where obstacles are thrown at me, I process what is going on and consider my options before choosing how to respond.

I put so much hard work into preparing for that charity fight, but I had to take a job abroad in the middle of my training. It wasn't the ideal fit with what I was trying to achieve in the boxing ring, as the job was very social and there would be lots of late-evening drinking involved. I had choices to make, but I took the discipline I had learned from boxing with me and chose not to drink. It might have been nice to have a few drinks with everyone, but I respected myself and the work I had been doing with Gary too much to let that slip. Knowing that going backwards with my training would be a disservice to what Gary and I had achieved so far, I stayed away from the booze-filled nights and hungover days. I also knew that if I lost the fight, I would always wonder if I would have won it if I had taken a different approach to that time abroad.

It was my first real experience of long-term discipline when it came to achieving a physical goal, and I've used this same approach in every subsequent challenge because, quite simply, it works. I entered that ring knowing I had committed everything to training for the fight. I had brought all of me into the process, with nothing holding me back. Because of this approach, I was rewarded, won all three rounds, and helped raise money for a deserving cause. Whether I won or lost didn't even matter, because I knew I had put every single part of myself into it. I could climb into that ring with my head held high.

Learning how to box turned out to be my saviour. At the time, I didn't think I wanted to learn a new skill or leave my comfort zone, but it turned out that this was exactly what I needed. That's the thing about leaving what we know – what is comfortable – we learn new skills and have new experiences, which will often aid us in other situations. For me, finding Gary and learning how to box improved my approach in all my subsequent challenges, and I would never have experienced that unless I was prepared to leave the comfort of what I knew.

Lesson 51: If You Don't Know, Don't Worry

Even when we've made the brave decision to leave the comfort of what we know and try something new, we can often end up sprinting back to that safe place when things get too challenging. Facing something new can be overwhelming; it can feel like the hurdles in front of us are insurmountable. Once that initial doubt begins to creep in, we might start building further barriers in our minds: we're too old, we're too young, we've missed our chance, no one will take us seriously . . . The list of reasons not to do something could fill a book when they're fuelled by an anxious mind.

Part of my work involves mentoring people when they approach me for help with their running challenges. People started to approach me after the patio runs, and this was pretty surreal as I hadn't been running seriously for that long. When they come to me, they are willing to commit themselves to the cause but sometimes still have one foot in their old life, ready to bolt back to it. They believe there is so much they don't know about pace, nutrition and training that it couldn't possibly work. They carefully explain all the things they don't know and what they haven't done before. Their anxiety clearly mounts as they continue, and they've practically talked themselves out of it before I can reassure them that what they are feeling is entirely normal.

What I tell them is always the same. It doesn't matter how long you have been doing something, there will always be more to learn, and you only learn by doing it. Rather than worrying about what you don't know, focus on what you do. Then, lean on those around you with more experience in those areas for advice, and decide whether that advice works for you. But you will only know this for sure when you start putting that advice into practice, because what works for one person might not work for the next. A certain method or approach might not suit your body type, personality, other commitments or budget.

Whenever someone asks me for advice about running shoes, nutrition or performance, I always make it clear that I can only advise them on what works for me. It's important to be open about these things, and I will never preach that my approach is the Holy Gospel. Instead, it's a potential approach that they can trial to see if it works for them too. What can be really effective for one person can be completely ineffective for another, but that doesn't mean you should give up. More research will be needed, and following different advice can provide that moment of realization that you've found the approach that works for you.

It can be easy to think that we must accumulate a stack of knowledge of how to do something before attempting it ourselves. But this often means we miss out on the valuable experience of doing it, which can teach us so much more. The order of learning is back to front. Once you have achieved one thing, run one race, painted one picture or secured your first customer, you will have banked a certain amount of knowledge. You then move forward from that point and repeat, pushing to level your knowledge up, again and again, gathering experience along the way.

We so often put people on pedestals. But these people are not impossibly high up above us – they're just further ahead. My dad has generated everything he has by learning on the job. It's the approach he takes with everything in his life, from building his successful business with my mum to deciding to build an extension on our house, which he did all by himself. He has learned everything through the experience of doing it, and I look up to him so much for that.

The other thing to remember about these high-achieving people is that they aren't winning every week. They will have times when they run a race, enter a negotiation or give a speech, and don't perform as well as they had hoped. They can be one of the best at what they do, but that doesn't mean their formula works every time. Life can be unpredictable, and the most minor change can mean a winning formula isn't suitable for that situation. But high achievers learn from these experiences and adjust their approach. Through this process of gaining experience and learning from it, they innovate and potentially make huge leaps forward.

Instead of being anxious about the unknown, we could try to flip that anxiety into excitement. Physiologically, they're really similar feelings, as they both usually involve a higher heart rate, sweating more, and that feeling of butterflies in your stomach; and we have the power to transform them. We can convert that anxious energy into something useful. Instead of thinking 'I don't know anything', reframe it as 'I'm going to learn so much'.

Rather than trying to accumulate all the answers, we should perhaps enjoy the process of progressive learning. One of the benefits of being outside of a formal education system is that you have the autonomy and ability to tailor how you absorb knowledge and who you go to for advice. You no longer have to follow a set curriculum – you can make your own. Some of the greatest runners I know are in their fifties. Physically, they might not be as fast as they once were, but they have accumulated years of knowledge and know there is still more to learn. The very fact that they're still running ultra-marathons is the sign of a great and successful runner to me.

You also have the choice to be patient with yourself and the process because you are setting the standards and the time frame. It's okay not to know something – you can just give it a go. You have the rest of your life to work it out.

Lesson 52: Don't Let Imposter Syndrome Hold You Back

'Who the hell am I to do the warm-up for 20,000 runners?'

This was my exact thought when I received a request from a company to motivate and warm up the huge 10k run they host every year. That thought was imposter syndrome creeping in. I had to remind myself that they'd asked me because I had run 76 marathons in 76 days, and set a new world record. I had earned the right to be asked, but my imposter syndrome was still there discrediting what I had achieved.

When I was thinking about this chapter, I had initially called it 'Overcome Imposter Syndrome', but that makes it sound like once we've overcome imposter syndrome in one situation, it is done with. This isn't how imposter syndrome works, as it will often resurface. If we keep pushing the boundaries of what we can achieve, we will keep entering places where we haven't always belonged. Therefore, we might never overcome imposter syndrome because we keep stretching our accomplishments and finding ourselves among new peers. But that's not important. What is important is that we don't let imposter syndrome hold us back.

When we push ourselves to achieve our goals, people

are more likely to notice what we are doing. There might even be some independent recognition of what we have accomplished. It's easy to look around us and think there are people out there who are better than us or more deserving. But we need to take the mental step of recognizing that we belong in the space we are occupying, and that what we have done is worthy of recognition.

At the root of imposter syndrome is often a fear of feeling shame. We are scared of opening ourselves up to the possibility of being rejected, laughed at or not taken seriously. Shame is a powerful deterrent when it comes to allowing what we do to be viewed or judged. In my experience, the feeling of imposter syndrome is often a learned behaviour that comes from a lifetime of the reactions and influence of others. But while we don't have any control over what others think about us, we can control how we react. Celebrating other people's achievements sets the tone for the reaction we expect when we tackle or complete something ourselves.

The running community has been incredibly supportive of my work, and I've done everything I can to return that support because I firmly believe running should be open to everyone. It shouldn't be a place filled with judgement or elitism. When it comes to running challenges, many people are scared to start them because of imposter syndrome. But a 24-hour run or 250k ultramarathon is such a unique experience that it will completely change your mindset about what is possible. Most people will straight away say, 'Oh no, I could never do that.' But when I ask them why they can't do it, they don't really have an answer. They just firmly believe they don't have the ability. That's imposter syndrome.

I've seen people from all walks of life achieve both of those runs — all different sizes, abilities and ages. They might not manage it in the fastest time in the world, but they still completed it. Removing the competition element lessens the pressure, which reduces the chance of imposter syndrome rising up.

People often face imposter syndrome in their careers as well. They feel held back in the job they are in but also don't have the confidence to make a change.

The more you work on imposter syndrome, the less hold it has on you. It is by facing your fears that you overcome them. Only by completing something, or at least learning from the experience, will you have something to fight back with.

The first step to ensuring that imposter syndrome doesn't hold you back is to look at your progression and what you have already achieved, and we'll be covering that in the next chapter.

Lesson 53: Look at How Far You've Come

I was speaking with someone at my gym recently who was telling me that she still wasn't improving in the functional fitness classes she was taking three times a week. She saw herself as someone dripping in sweat and unable to keep up with the rest of the class. This didn't ring true for me, as I remembered when she first joined the gym six months ago she had struggled to do a single class. I reminded her of this and asked what she would have thought if I had told her then that she would be religiously attending three classes a week? She admitted that she wouldn't have thought it possible because her lifestyle outside the gym would have got in the way. But she had made those changes, reduced her drinking and changed her eating to get to where she was now. There was a ladder of progression, and the evidence was clear – for her to be able to take three classes a week, at the very least, her stamina was building. Rather than looking at her performance in the class in isolation and using that as evidence that she was not improving, I nudged her to focus on all the progress she had made that enabled her to attend three classes a week.

Would I have been able to jump straight into running 76 marathons in 76 days without my own ladder of progression? Of course not. It's likely I would have seriously injured myself within the first few weeks. It was my progression that made it possible. A wheelchair marathon in Berlin, John O'Groats to Land's End, my patio marathons, running marathons in four nations in twenty-four hours and Sri Lanka were all part of the progression towards the 76 Marathons. When my anxiety tries to weaken me, I can now look back over the past few years and what I have accomplished. Whenever my imposter syndrome says I can't do something or don't belong, I have plenty of evidence to prove it is wrong.

Taking the time to look at our progression is essential. When we begin setting ourselves challenges and goals, it is very easy to constantly live for the future. Our mind settles on a place far away and barely recognizes or celebrates the steps we are taking to reach that place. Once we finally arrive at that achievement, we are already setting ourselves a new task without registering how far we have come. Without allowing ourselves time to reflect on our journey, the destination we want to reach will just continue to get further away. We will feel exhausted and disappointed for never reaching it, rather than feeling the fulfilment of having hit lots of targets along the way.

I've been guilty of doing this. But the stress fracture in my foot from the 76 Marathons forced me to stop and take a break. I couldn't train properly without causing permanent damage so, finally, I had time to process what I had been through. When I was in the middle of the marathons, everything was a bit of a blur because

I was so focused on putting one foot in front of another and just getting through each day. Every morning I would get up and have a new finish line to focus on. There was no time to dwell on what had happened the day before or reflect on things. Of course, there were moments of clarity where a particular story from another runner or a beautiful bit of scenery broke through the fog in my brain, but it was only after resting for a while that I could access all those memories that my brain had filed away but never reviewed.

It was a form of closure, and it also allowed me to celebrate the small wins that added up to something much greater. If we don't acknowledge the journey, then what do we do it all for? Whether it's facing a tough meeting at work, ticking off a to-do list or beating a personal best, we need to savour those moments. They are just as important as the big wins in life, and that is what makes life worth living.

Allowing ourselves time to appreciate our progression provides us with the clarity and mental space to ask the question 'What's next?'

Lesson 54: Someone is Always Rooting for You

We've all probably had at least one time where we can't believe where life has taken us. Marathon 30, in Liverpool, was exactly one of those times. Chris Taylor had just told me that it had been arranged for us to run around the pitch at Anfield, and I couldn't believe the club had given me this honour. Running around the ground of one of the greatest football teams in the world is something I will never forget. An impossibility that became a reality.

My love for Liverpool Football Club started at a very young age, and it was influenced by a very important woman who played a massive part in my childhood. I first met Betty after she had moved to our area and was looking for some work. My dad asked her to help around the house for a few hours a week, but he soon realized the house wasn't really her priority. My sister and I were. We became Betty's adopted grandchildren, whom she adored, and we loved her too. She was the only person I know who could get away with telling my dad to sod off when he asked her to do some work. After a few weeks, the banter between them put a smile on all our faces. Betty would spend more and more time with us, and looked after my sister and me when our parents went out. We'd often watch Liverpool play on the television together. I didn't think much about her enthusiasm for football at the time other than how much she adored her team. Her passion for Liverpool was so infectious that it would eventually pass on to me, and it has remained with me since.

A few years later, my mum told me that Betty wasn't well. I went to visit her and barely recognized the person in front of me as she was so frail. I couldn't understand what illness could do this to her. It turned out she had cancer, something my parents had decided to keep from my sister and me with good intentions. One evening, we got the call to tell us that Betty had passed away. The news devastated the entire family. It felt as if it had only been a few days ago that she had been sitting at our kitchen table eating her packed lunch. She left a hole in our family that could never be filled. Supporting Liverpool FC kept me close to her, as I knew it was something we could share even though she was no longer with us.

Walking through the tunnel at Anfield during Marathon 30, I stared up at the sky with the biggest grin as I knew Betty would be looking down at me and laughing. This was our moment to share. I stuck my earphones in and played 'You'll Never Walk Alone' on repeat. I couldn't stop thinking about Betty and how this young lad from Lincolnshire who had watched his team on the screen was now running around that iconic ground twenty years later. Even though I was running in an empty stadium, it felt as though every single seat was filled.

That ethos of 'You'll Never Walk Alone' has stuck with me since I first heard the Liverpool fans singing it. Over the years I have come up with lots of creative and daring ideas that most people have advised me not to do, but I have always found one person who will support me and walk alongside me. Usually, once that happens, it snowballs and more step forward.

We can be that person for others as well. I have a friend who dreamed of running a kilometre to honour every man who died by suicide each week for a year, amounting to a heart-breaking 84 kilometres a week. He came to me with the idea, and my response was: 'Do it. This is your calling. You've got the mental strength for this, and I can introduce you to people who can help with the physical side.' He made a huge success of it, left a job he didn't enjoy, and created a new life centred around his purpose, putting himself on a path that fulfilled him.

You might feel like no one believes in or is invested in what you are doing, but I want to reassure you that it's not the reality. Even if someone you've spoken to isn't rooting for you, it doesn't mean they're not invested in you as an individual. They just don't share your interests or don't have the capacity to support you at that time.

This might initially be disappointing, but there is a silver lining to us all having different interests. Because for every person who doesn't support your ambitions, there will be plenty more who will. If you look on social media, there are a legion of fans and enthusiastic followers for some of the most niche interests. There might be hundreds or even thousands of people who would cheer you on, because they share those same beliefs or passions. You just haven't met them yet. There are whole communities of people who would be the first to jump up and say, 'Do it. This is your calling.'

You could try to find them, or continue on your path with just the knowledge that they are out there. The choice is yours, as only you know how important this is to you in completing your mission. Whether you decide to connect with them or not, you will never walk alone.

Lesson 55: Wake Up with a Smile and an Open Mind

Around seven years ago, I was at a party and met an Aussie lad called Zac White. We hit it off straight away, and spent the entire night drinking together and discussing the adventures we wanted to go on. He was part of a group called the Neverland Boys, who had created a life out of travelling on a shoestring budget and creating content out of it. They would visit a country, create unbelievable content, and offer it to companies who, in return, would help fund their trips. It was pure freedom, based on a stripped-back lifestyle where only the essentials were needed to create the most incredible experiences.

I had grown up in Lincolnshire and spent what felt like half my childhood aimlessly wandering around the countryside, so this adventurous lifestyle greatly appealed to me. It felt like meeting Zac and hearing about his completely different approach to life was exactly what I needed. I'd been in a funk for a while after a relationship had ended and wasn't satisfied with what I was doing with my time. Zac was full of enthusiasm for life, and just being in his company for an evening made me feel more optimistic about the changes I could make.

The next day, I was surprised when Zac messaged me

and said he was heading to Greece for ten days to travel around five islands. He wanted to know whether I wanted to join him and the other Neverland Boys on the trip. At first, I wasn't too sure. How many times do you meet someone when you're drunk and think they're your new best friend or business partner, only to realize the next day that you can't even remember what you were talking about? But I was going through a tricky time with my career and had just broken up with my girlfriend, and there didn't seem to be much stopping me. In the end, I thought, 'Why not?' I was twenty-six, responsibility-free, and I wanted to sample a different way of life.

So I booked a flight and flew to Athens, where I met the rest of the Neverland Boys. At that time in my life I was surrounded by a lot of materialism and felt quite lost in that environment. It was exciting to leave that behind and try something new.

Every morning, we would wake up and create something from nothing. One day, we got up really early to do some cliff jumping at a beautiful spot on a Greek island. Some yachts were close by, and the boys started filming themselves flipping off the side of a yacht. One of the yacht owners suddenly emerged and shouted at us about what we were doing. Completely unfazed, Zac swam over to him and explained about their work and what they were doing there. The owner asked him if he had ever filmed on a boat before, and Zac explained that he had done it several times and showed him some footage.

It turned out that the man wasn't just the owner of

the boat he was standing on – he owned a whole fleet. Impressed by the content they were producing, he told Zac that he could take his pick of boats for the day. Zac had created something from nothing – just by waking up with a smile and an open mind.

At that time, I was uneasy about the direction my life was taking, and what Zac and his friends had going on was the antidote I needed. That trip showed me how valuable the right environment can be. It wasn't about alcohol, spending money, getting into the best parties, or paying thousands for a table at a nightclub or restaurant. Instead, we had the bare minimum on a beach. The simplicity of the trip was a breath of fresh air. Every morning, I would wake up with a smile because of the people I was with and the things I was doing.

When the trip ended, I took that newfound enthusiasm back home with me, relieved that my dissatisfaction with my life wasn't because something was wrong with me; it was because I didn't feel fulfilled. I stripped everything in my life back as much as I could. Because of Zac and his friends, I now try to approach each day with a smile on my face and an open mind. It is amazing where those two things can take you.

Lesson 56: It's Not About What You Have, but What You Do with It

I'm very fortunate that I come from a privileged background because of the business my mum and dad built together. It would be dishonest to try to downplay that and the opportunities it has opened up for me. Because of the family I grew up in and the career that I ended up with, I've never had to worry about my education, paying the rent or feeding my family, like my dad did when he was younger.

Whenever I'm doing a challenge, the media always raise the fact of my privileged background and expect me to comment on it. I'm left wondering, 'What is the question here?' It doesn't make sense to me that I am being asked to comment on my background. I could understand it if I had the ability, resources and network to help others but was choosing not to. But when someone is trying to utilize what they have to help others, I don't really understand why they must be questioned about it.

Ultimately, we can't help which family we are born into. None of us can. When it comes to my situation, I've tried to make it clear that I'm committed to using my platform to help as many people as possible. There are far more fun and less painful options that I could have chosen. I don't consider myself materialistic; I don't showcase a life of luxury or talk about what I've bought. That doesn't appeal to me because I know it doesn't fulfil me. What does fulfil me is a simpler life where I spend as much time as I can outdoors, preferably with my family and friends, and support as many people as possible by testing my mental and physical strength. Yes, my background has made that more accessible for me, and I am fully aware of that. But I can't erase that background. All I can do is decide what I do with it.

I also take this approach with the people I meet. I try not to judge them on their background, but instead look at what they do with their lives now. What have they set themselves to achieve? Who do they help? How do they approach life? All of this is what informs my opinion of a person. It doesn't have to mean grand gestures or life-consuming challenges, as we can't all be expected to do that. It's simply about how much someone puts back into the world compared to how much they take out.

Lesson 57: Focus on Progress Rather Than Perfection

Whenever I finish up a longer challenge, I have several weeks where I eat exactly what I want. It's a time to relax and eat whatever takes my fancy, and I don't put any restrictions on my diet. But after a few weeks of this, I'll return to healthier eating. I'll still slip up and overindulge occasionally, but the next day I'll go back to what I should be eating. One slip-up doesn't mean that I throw in the towel. When I take a step backwards, as long as I return to the right food, I am still making progress in the right direction. This can apply to whatever we are working towards, whether it's related to running, a personal best, losing weight or improving a relationship or something at work.

Too often, we focus on the bigger picture, which tends to be the end goal. But what is actually really important is the process by which we achieve it. The small accomplishments amount to the bigger picture, but they are also an education within themselves. You will make mistakes on the way to your goal, and learn from the process. We tend to belittle those moments when, actually, they are where we validate ourselves. We need to acknowledge what we have accomplished every step of the way rather than waiting until the end to have a huge celebration. Because the smaller moments need celebrating too.

We are also never the finished model, because there is no such thing. We are constantly evolving, and therefore should cherish the incremental steps made along the way. When I'm preparing for a challenge, I don't focus on the run itself; I focus on the process leading up to it. That is the primary focus, and is where sacrifices and willpower are required. The fact that I am able to step onto the start line is the reward for all that hard work. The problem with just focusing on achieving the perfect outcome is that if things don't turn out how you hoped they would, where does that leave all your hard work? Is it null and void?

We can also become fixated on the size of what we set ourselves and how much success others are having. We can look at someone running 250 kilometres in a week, view that as the perfect result, and wonder what the point is in our 5k run. Or we can see how much money someone is making in their business at twenty-five years old and decide there is no point in us setting up our own because we're twenty years older than them and missed our chance.

For me, there was a natural progression to the 76 Marathons, and it took six years to get to that point. The size of each challenge increased, and with it, so did my physical and mental resilience. Thousands of tiny accomplishments along the way led to the opportunity and ability to run so many marathons around the UK.

I didn't know six years ago that this is what it would culminate in when all that progress was put in place.

Striving for 'perfection' is ultimately unrewarding as it doesn't really exist. There is no real end destination, as perfection is subjective and will differ between people. When we concentrate on progress, we can enjoy the journey, forgive ourselves our occasional blips, take an overview of what we've achieved and use this to motivate us to achieve more. With perfection, we will probably never reach that destination and will spend our lives striving for it but never satisfied. That's why I believe in progress over perfection every time.

Lesson 58: Don't Sell Yourself Short

It is so incredibly easy to sell ourselves short. Even the best athletes do this, and I was reminded of this recently when I was chatting with Anya Culling, who had a remarkable journey into running. We were sitting in the office when she told me that her marathon time hadn't progressed as she had hoped in the last couple of months, which was beginning to concern her. She was even wondering if her sponsor would drop her. I had to smile as she told me that, as it was clear that she was selling herself short.

Anya had underestimated the impact she had on others and why she was sponsored in the first place. I leaned forward and told her that, with the greatest respect, she wasn't being sponsored because she could run a marathon in 2 hours and 34 minutes. She was being sponsored because of the person she was and the journey she was on. In only four years, she had gone from running the London Marathon in 4 hours and 34 minutes to slicing two hours off her time and now running for England. At nineteen, she had run for fun. At twenty-three, she was representing her country alongside England's best athletes.

When you step back and look at the whole picture of

what Anya achieved in such a short time, it is absolutely mind-blowing, but her view was clouded by the most recent month or two. She was selling herself short because she had so much more to give than an elite marathon time of 2 hours and 34 minutes. She was already inspiring other women and men to hope that they could also achieve something remarkable. Anya hadn't run in school or joined a running club at a young age. She only started training and learning to run properly after her first marathon. During the COVID-19 lockdowns, Anya began to run most days and taught herself the physical and mental requirements for long-distance running. She managed this incredible achievement through pure hard work.

She met her future running coach in a park just by chance, and her life took another turn into the world of professional running and coaching. The people she started training didn't necessarily want to run for England or complete a marathon in two and a half hours. They were inspired by what she had achieved through determination, commitment and consistency. That was what made her unique, and reconnecting with that person who loved what she was doing would mean that she would feel fulfilled by her passion and see every day as an accomplishment.

We all need to remind ourselves to not sell ourselves short. I have come away from a couple of challenges feeling a bit deflated that the media didn't pick up on it and wondering how much more money we could have raised if there had been more publicity. But that approach undermines the impact of the challenge and the connection I made with people along the way.

When we sell ourselves short, we are often looking for external validation that what we are doing is worthwhile. When I fall into this trap now, I remind myself to take a step back and readjust my viewpoint and consider every part of my journey. It is the story of our life so far that provides this validation, not the current situation.

Lesson 59: Regret Will Outlast Momentary Pain

The start of the Berlin Marathon with Tano did not go as smoothly as we had hoped. It was 2018, and after months of training in our wheelchairs, we had finally made it to the start line with our families watching from the sidelines. As we pushed our way towards the official in charge to sign in, one side of my wheelchair deflated. I had a puncture. Worse still, I didn't have a spare tyre or inner tubing to replace it with.

For months, I hadn't had a single problem with the wheelchair I'd used every day, and on the very morning of the race my tyre was flat. In only a few seconds, I had gone from absolute elation at being able to support Tano in achieving his goal to utter despair that I wouldn't be able to compete with him. Tano was going to have to do this alone.

In a last-ditch effort, I approached other participants to ask if they had a spare tyre or inner tubing. No one did, but I kept going down the line, speaking with officials, participants, and anyone who might possibly be able to help. On the brink of giving up, I returned to my wheelchair. But at the very moment I was about to retire, a repair kit team emerged from the crowd. They had the correct tubing, so they got to work, and in ten minutes they had managed to repair the tyre. Tano and I grinned at each other and rolled our way towards the official to finally sign in.

A woman with a lanyard came over to inspect our wheelchairs. She confirmed that everything was okay but said, 'Can I just check the helmets you are both going to be wearing?' Tano and I glanced at each other. We didn't have helmets. Apparently, it was mandatory to have a helmet when racing in a wheelchair, for health-and-safety reasons. My mouth went dry as I explained that we didn't have them and weren't even aware of the requirement. She was sympathetic to our situation but added it was in the information sent to us ahead of the race. She kindly said she would speak to someone but finished with: 'But it's not looking good.'

Five minutes later, she returned with her superior, who point blank refused to let us race without helmets. The supervisor wouldn't even entertain the thought of it. No helmet, no race. We were screwed.

The race was starting soon, and we had to leave with one of the waves of wheelchair racers. I entered panic mode and began calling all my friends and family who had come to support us. I told them to spread out across Berlin to find a cycle shop and either buy us two helmets or find someone who would lend them to us.

While this was all going on, we were being filmed for a documentary we were making about the challenge. Our setbacks would make great viewing, but I knew that if we didn't find the two helmets soon, the challenge would be over before it had even begun. I told the videographer to stay with Tano, and began running through the streets of Berlin to find two helmets. I stopped countless cyclists on the road but had no luck, as either they didn't speak English or understandably didn't want to give their helmets to a stranger. Looking at my watch, I realized we had missed the start time for the first wave, which included some of the wheelchair users competing in the marathon. I felt sick – I had no idea if we would make it in time for the next wave, but all I could do was carry on searching.

After running around Berlin for about an hour, I still didn't have the helmets, and I knew I'd soon have to return empty-handed. At that moment, I received a call from my mum, who told me to meet her at a checkpoint as she had managed to pull off a miracle. She had approached a couple cycling together and pleaded with them to lend their helmets to us. This couple must have realized my mum was a low flight risk, so they very generously agreed to lend their helmets to us for the day. My mum took their address and promised to return them.

By the time I got back to Tano with the helmets, I was drenched in sweat, having run close to 10 kilometres around Berlin. My stress levels were also beyond anything I'd experienced before. It was then that Tano quietly told me that the last wave had already gone. After months of training and preparation, we had missed the race. We had fallen at the first hurdle. I was distraught.

As we tried to absorb what this meant, the female

official who had first approached us about our helmets rushed over. She explained she'd managed to pull some strings, and if we left right now before the elite runners set off, they would let us compete.

Rushing to put on our borrowed helmets, I scrambled around for everything I would need for the race. I wasn't mentally ready and was already exhausted after my unexpected morning run. It was my first-ever marathon. I was doing it in a wheelchair, and I felt utterly unprepared. But we just had to get on with it. I knew that the feeling of regret if we gave up now would long outlast the momentary pain I was faced with.

We pushed our way to the start line. The elite runners kindly lifted us up to pass us to the front so we could set off before them. There was no ceremony for us starting the race; one of the officials just yelled 'Go!' at Tano and me, and off we went. For 3 kilometres, it was just Tano and I wheeling our way through the streets of Berlin with a German crowd cheering us along. We looked at each other as the crowd clapped for the two lone competitors in wheelchairs – we'd done it.

Way behind us, the elite runners set off. There was an extraordinary moment when Tano and I were pushing ourselves along, and one of the greatest marathon runners of our time, Eliud Kipchoge, ran past with his entourage of other runners. We looked on in awe as they streaked ahead. We later discovered that Kipchoge had set a new world record for the fastest marathon time: 2 hours, 1 minute and 39 seconds. History was made that day.

Tano and I had faced a choice when our morning didn't go as planned. We could have crumbled and accepted that we wouldn't race that day because the world seemed to have gone against us in every way. But instead we decided to go through the momentary pain of fighting for what we wanted.

That lesson I learned in Berlin is one that I have carried with me through every challenge – and painful moment – since. Whether it is physical or emotional pain, that short-term sacrifice is worth it to avoid the feeling of regret that can hang over you forever.

The pain and sacrifices we go through to achieve our goals won't last forever, but the pride from accomplishing them will.

Lesson 60: You Can Do It, You've Just Not Done It Yet

No matter how dedicated we are to something, life can often get in the way and change things out of our control. When I began training for the 76 Marathons, I had no idea that most of the world would be in lockdown because of COVID-19 within a few months. My training had to be put on hold because we weren't allowed outside for more than an hour at a time and I needed to practise running for much longer than that. There was nothing I could do about it, so I turned my attention to the marathons around my patio instead, which was something that was within my control.

As is often the case, life had taken me in a different direction than expected, and as the months passed, I talked myself out of attempting to run a marathon in every city in the UK. I decided running all those marathons was a great idea, but it simply wasn't possible consecutively. No one had done it before because it was a logistical nightmare, combined with the constant physical and mental exertion. I had let life get in the way and convince me to give up on an idea that I had once been so passionate about.

I moved on to my new priority: running an ultra-marathon in Sri Lanka. Running for five days in extreme conditions on zero sleep while incredibly dehydrated was psychologically one of the most challenging things I've done. I had to force my mind to new depths to find the strength to get through it, and by the end I knew that whether it was 250 kilometres or 76 marathons, I had the mindset to do it. Pushing myself to those lengths gave me a renewed focus to make the 76 happen, and I knew that if I didn't try, I would regret it for the rest of my life.

More than three years would pass from when the idea was first conceived to when I set my foot on the start line for the first marathon, in Inverness. In the time that had passed, seven towns were turned into cities following the Queen's Jubilee. So what had originally been conceived as 69 marathons turned into 76. By the time I crossed the finish line in London after eleven weeks of running marathons and completing the dream I had been chasing for years, I realized that when we are passionate about doing something and life is getting in the way, we shouldn't say we can't do something – we just haven't done it yet.

That change in mindset is a potent one. It removes many of the barriers in our minds about what we are capable of. Saying we haven't done something *yet* allows the possibility to remain on the table. It hasn't been swept to the floor for someone else to pick up. When we repeatedly tell ourselves that we can't do something, it sends a negative signal through our mind that constantly reinforces that it's not a possibility. We prove to ourselves that we can't do it by not doing it.

Adjusting your mindset doesn't mean you have to complete what you set yourself within a week or even a year. It could take you ten years – it took me six years to get to the point where I successfully completed the 76 Marathons. But saying that you haven't done it yet removes the all-or-nothing approach of either doing it now or never doing it at all. Circumstances and life might get in the way, and that's completely normal. It's better to delay than remove it as a possibility.

This mindset will also help when you attempt something and don't achieve it first time. When I started seriously thinking about the 76 Marathons, I immediately knew it would be an inspiring challenge, so I set myself the most ambitious fundraising target I could think of. My previous challenges had raised around £25,000 each for charity, but this time, I wanted to smash that target. So I set myself the goal of raising £1 million. I have always wanted to raise a million pounds for charity, and I decided I might as well attempt that in one challenge. It was ambitious, but I needed that pressure to motivate me.

By the time all the donations had come in, I had raised £400,000, far exceeding anything I had raised before in a single challenge. It wasn't the £1 million I had wanted, but I gave every single ounce of myself to that challenge. There was nothing more I could have put into it, so I knew I could still hold my head high. If you've given it everything, what is there to be disappointed in?

Ultimately, some things in life are outside your control, but that doesn't mean you won't achieve them eventually. It just means that, at that time, it unfortunately didn't work out. I'm disappointed we didn't raise more money, as it would have helped more people, but I'm not disappointed in myself because I gave everything I could to the process. And that outcome gave me an incentive to continue with my work until the day I successfully raise the full £1 million for charity. It might take one, two, three or even ten more challenges to fulfil that dream, but I know it is achievable if I keep giving all of myself to them.

When it comes to raising £1 million for charity, it isn't a case of *if* I will do it – it is *when* I will do it.

Lesson 61: Be Proactive Rather Than Reactive

Around a year ago, it had gotten to the point that regular pain from injuries had become such an ordinary feeling for me that I had become complacent. Because I was doing so many challenges, I had accepted discomfort as part of my life. I remember waking up one morning and realizing that this was self-inflicted and therefore could be improved – it did not need to be this way. As far as I could see, no one else running distances like me was in a similar situation; they weren't talking about the pain they were in every day. Why was I choosing to wake up sore, tired and uneasy? It was clear something needed to change.

I started focusing a lot more on maintenance and recovery. I would see a physio and soft-tissue therapist every week, and during the sessions I would ask them about the best ways to maintain my health. Across the board, they would tell me that their biggest concern is that people only come to see them when something is wrong, when they should have been having appointments throughout the year to *prevent* something from going wrong. We work so hard to test ourselves and build our bodies up, but so few of us will invest the time or money to counter that with the necessary rehab or physio.

This changed my viewpoint on my own health. I'm

incredibly fortunate to have been gifted a functional body, and it belittles that gift if I don't do what is within my means to help maintain its functionality.

The longer we leave something, the harder it is to do anything about it. If I've had a poor night's sleep, I can wake up feeling quite jaded. Even though it's the last thing I want to do, I'll get into an ice-cold plunge pool and instantly feel better. I have a daily choice to make: I can feel tired, muggy and sore for most of the day, or I can go into an ice plunge for two minutes and come out feeling genuinely replenished with a positive mindset. If I do that most days, no matter how I'm feeling that morning, its impact on the quality of my life will be immeasurable.

It's the same with our mental health. We need to find small ways of supporting it each day – of doing the things that make us feel calm, content and in control. For me, it is ensuring that I exercise somehow each day, even if it's just going for a brief run, and of course a dunk in the ice bath helps me as well. Just like our physical health, our mental well-being won't be there for us for the rest of our lives if we don't tend to it.

If you had asked me ten or fifteen years ago what I valued the most, my answer would have been very different to the one I have now. It is only when you begin to witness mortality or serious illnesses that you realize how finite this life is. I recently lost a family member to a heart condition, and we found out that another relative had the same condition. A lot of the family have now been tested to see if they have the condition too. If that's the case, they can put steps in place to ease the strain on their heart. This is still a reactive decision, though. A proactive approach to my health is making the decisions each day that I know will benefit me both mentally and physically. Consistency with my sleep, nutrition, hydration, recovery, strength and mobility is key.

When we're younger, we know we won't always be here, but the implications of that don't quite sink in. Seeing just how short life can be has helped to reverse my approach to my mental and physical health, and preventative treatment is now what I spend the most money on out of all my outgoings. My long-term health is my biggest priority, as I want to ensure I'm as healthy and active as possible for my daughter. I want to continue doing what I love and be able to function freely every day.

Whether it is changing careers, starting a new relationship, finding a new hobby or building a business, the proactive decisions we make increase our chances of success. When we take action proactively, it comes from a place of thoughtfulness and preparation. We are ahead of the curve and have considered all possibilities. When we take action reactively, we are often on the back foot, having to make decisions quickly with little capacity to review everything necessary to make the best choice. Whatever area of our life it relates to, proactiveness comes from a place of preparation, while reaction relies largely on an emotional response. Let's create the future we want rather than reacting to one we don't.

Lesson 62: Try to View Things from Other People's Perspective

With every experience comes a new opportunity to learn, and preparing for the Berlin Marathon and John O'Groats to Land's End challenge in a wheelchair were eye-opening experiences as they allowed me to view the world from someone else's perspective. I was doing them for my best mate Tano after he lost the use of his legs in an accident, and I knew that to make the most significant possible impact for the spinal injury community, raising money would not be enough. I wanted to try to understand the daily struggles they faced and what could be done to help with these.

For wheelchair users, the equipment, environment and support they need to function are massive factors in their day. I decided that training in a wheelchair would not be enough and that I would commute to work in my chair and integrate using it into my daily life. When faced with a hurdle in my wheelchair, I would have to find a solution to resolve it rather than taking the obvious route out.

It became clear that there were so many things in my life that I had taken for granted. I remember battling with a kerb for what felt like a lifetime. I could not get over it, but I eventually figured out how to achieve this.

I'm not saying that I now understand what it's like to be permanently in a wheelchair, but it did give me a glimpse of a different perspective that I hadn't even been able to contemplate before. It surprised me at times how there was a lack of empathy while I was trying to move around the streets. People would sometimes avoid making eye contact with me, as if I weren't there right in front of them. The experience made me even more determined to raise India to not focus on Uncle Tano's wheelchair but instead to just see Uncle Tano.

We are told from a young age that we should consider other people's viewpoints, but until this experience I don't think I'd ever understood the value of it. Over the past six years, I've learned the importance of exposing myself to new viewpoints and experiences, as this allows me to grow and adapt. If I was still the same person I was six years ago, I don't think I would have achieved half the things I have done. But I have tried to spend as much time as I can familiarizing myself with other people's realities so that I can support them, and myself, as best as I can. Even when we discover a new way of doing things, it doesn't necessarily mean it is the right or only one. I try to be mindful when I give an opinion that I don't preach it as if it's the Holy Gospel. Although I can get excited about gaining a fresh perspective on something, what works for one person might not work for someone else, and each of us can only say what has helped us in our unique position.

We also have to be mindful that our experiences are

never the same as someone else's. I am incredibly aware of this when advocating for positive mental health because I have much easier access to help, such as therapy, than most people. Long NHS waiting lists mean that therapy isn't always an option for people who can't afford to pay for it, which is why I'm so determined to raise funds for the Samaritans and the work they do to support people who are really struggling. If we can try to understand a situation from as many people's perspectives as possible, we have a much better chance of connecting with them, supporting them and providing the best advice. It's about knowing the limitations of our understanding, and doing our best to educate ourselves.

Lesson 63: This Too Shall Pass

There will always be things that happen that are outside our control. A million different circumstances occur each day that can touch our lives either directly or indirectly. But as Marcus Aurelius said nearly 2,000 years ago, 'You have power over your mind – not outside events. Realize this, and you will find strength.' This quote resonates with me because, when we face adversity, we often feel powerless. We feel helpless and abandoned to circumstances we can't control. We might turn to others and hope that they will assist us, but actually the strength to change the impact of that situation can only come from within. This is because only we have the power to choose how we react to it.

One of the ways I have coped with adverse and testing situations is to remind myself that 'this too shall pass'. Whatever the emotion we are feeling, it helps to know it will pass into a different one. Whether good, bad, ugly or beautiful, we aren't stuck in one feeling. Even when I was much younger and went through unbelievably dark periods that lasted for years, they eventually passed. I made changes within myself, and my outside circumstances altered as well, and life shifted into easier times. Because of that experience, whenever I go through troublesome situations now, I know they will come to an end. It's a case of being patient with the process. We want immediate change, but some things need to unfold, and all we can do is hold on, make the best decisions we can at the time, and ride those circumstances out.

As surely as the bad times will pass, so will the good ones. We can try to cling to them or chase them, but they will also move away from us. This is why trying to lead a 'happy' life is so futile. Happiness comes and goes, and we can only really appreciate what true happiness feels like if we have also been through darker times. Happiness is also something that shall pass. It is not something that stays for long, because an outside circumstance will interrupt it. If happiness were a constant, it would begin to feel mundane. We would start chasing euphoria, wanting to get higher and higher and doing everything possible to achieve that. But euphoria passes too, and when it does, where would that leave us?

We can also dwell too much on previous happy times. We look to the past and wish to remain there. We want to return to a time when an experience, achievement or recognition made us feel good about ourselves. When I come out of a challenge, I always know that an inevitable dip will come. But if I remain in the past, looking back on a previous time, it takes my attention away from the present. I'm no longer fully conscious or appreciative of the time I have right now. It also removes my ability to believe that the best times could still be ahead. When that hope for the future is taken away, we don't implement the steps that could create future successes. So instead, I try to be grateful in the moment before focusing on what comes next.

I've learned that contentment and fulfilment are far more lasting than happiness. They require deeper groundwork, so that when something outside our control comes along, it is less likely to shake that solid foundation. They can't protect me from everything, but knowing that difficult times are never permanent always helps. Because this too shall pass.

Lesson 64: Adversity is Inevitable, but You Choose Your Own Narrative

A large part of my work is about changing how we perceive people with mental illness. I don't want to be known as 'Josh Patterson who had depression'. If I held on to the things I have been through, it's unlikely you would be reading this book, because my narrative would be very different. My story would be that I was Joshua Patterson, who came from a broken home, struggles with his mental health, is no longer with his child's mother and failed in business. If I chose to be the victim of that, I would put out a very different energy.

But I get to choose my narrative. I don't need to hide anything; instead, I reframe how it is presented. Nowadays, the first thing people talk to me about is usually my challenges. When they ask me about the 76 Marathons, they often ask which charity I was raising money for, and I explain that it was for a mental health charity. They usually want to know why a mental health charity is close to my heart, and I tell them that I struggle with anxiety and had depression in the past. Rather than talking about what led me to my darkest moments, I explain that I'm really fortunate to have supportive family members, friends and access to therapy, and I know that not everyone has that – so I want to help those who don't have the support they need to receive it, so they can go on to lead fulfilled lives. The person I'm talking to won't focus on the fact that I have anxiety. Instead, they accept anxiety as part of my story and see what I am doing with it. Perhaps it also gives them a chance to redefine their interpretation of anxiety and mental health conditions. Ultimately, it's how we choose to react to adversity that inspires people to think differently about how they face it too.

When I look at my own past, I wouldn't want someone else to face what I have, but I also realize that it has shaped me into the person I am today. It has given me the desire, willingness and openness to evolve, adapt, develop, and ultimately achieve what I have done. If none of those things had happened, would I be in the position I'm in today? The answer is, I don't know. But I highly doubt I would have travelled in this direction.

Everyone will face some degree of adversity in their life. The outcome will depend on the way they frame it. Whether we like it or not, adversity will change the course of our lives. But we still get to choose the narrative.

Lesson 65: Focus on Fulfilment

I was recently giving a talk to young adults in an inner-city school when one of them asked how much money I made. I suggested to him that he should be asking me whether I was fulfilled in what I was doing. I had to respect that he asked me, though, as I think we often want to know what people earn but don't ask. Having this conversation made me think about how we approach our careers. Too often we focus on the financial side. We want to earn more, sell more, be better. Often even if we reach the magic number we always thought we wanted to earn, it suddenly doesn't seem like enough and we set another target and chase after that. But if someone wakes up and absolutely loves what they're doing, that is far more beneficial to the overall quality of their life than how much more money they made this month. I've also realized that there is higher chance of money following if you find something that fulfils you. When you love what you do, you are more motivated to work at it.

I'm proud to see my business growing and that there is so much belief in it from others. With my overactive and easily distracted mind, I'm so grateful to be part of something I love doing. Me being in the office early is a testament to that and a clear sign of how much I enjoy my work. Since the early days of just Ben, Dom, Walter, Katie and I, we've had to change offices three times because of the increasing numbers of employees to match the company's growth. Being in that environment is infectious, and our success is down to the culture, passion and time every single person puts into the company.

I have grown so much because of Runna. When you have a group of people all focused on the same outcome, seismic changes can happen in a short amount of time. Our passion for helping runners achieve their goals, from their first 5k all the way up to 250-kilometre ultra-marathons, carries us through the day. We want to support people from any walk of life with their running. That core belief directs everything we do, from our pricing to making our running plans available worldwide, and we recently celebrated the milestone of selling plans in 180 countries. It feels like we are putting something back into the world, and I'm so grateful that I've found a career doing something I love.

Because of the fulfilment it brings me, it never feels like work. It is the journey that excites me, and I want to be present for that as much as I can.

Lesson 66: Children Can be
Our Greatest Teachers

When I found out I was going to be a father, a huge range of feelings crashed over me. The first one that came to the surface, and which remained there for some time, was that I was too young and wasn't ready or prepared for this next stage in my life. Ultimately, I was scared. My life felt unsettled, and I was unsure of what I could offer to my child. I had always imagined that being a father was still far off in the future, and I would have more experiences to prepare me, but that's not how life works. We won't always have time to prepare for everything. Instead, we have to step up when we're needed. These unexpected experiences force our hand, make us show what we are made of, and the result can be life-changing.

Now, whenever I'm faced with a situation where the challenge seems too great, I look back at how I approached becoming a dad. Although it was scary at first, I adapted my life to work with India in it. I had initially worried that looking after her would place a limitation on what I could do and affect my training, but I found ways around it. I would put India in her buggy on a Saturday and take her for a run with me, and she loved it. People often talk about the limitations that come with being a parent, but I have tried to integrate India into whatever it is that I'm doing. Whether she remembers it or not, I have wanted her to be a part of everything in my life. For a couple of years, I trained for challenges with her in a buggy, and I have so many fond memories of that time we spent together preparing for me to achieve some of my ambitions. I didn't want it to be the case that one minute I was a dad, the next I was training for a challenge, and then back to being a dad again. I didn't like the idea of that separation.

Six years later, I know I have fulfilled that role in the best way I can. I have given it everything I've got and learned more along the way, and will keep adapting to meet my daughter's ever-evolving needs. I look at the person she has grown into and feel immense pride that she is happy, loving, nurturing, ambitious and funny. What's even more incredible is that she has taught me so much about myself. Before I had India my biggest fear in life had always been love. This doesn't come from wanting to live a single lifestyle but instead from wanting to protect myself from being hurt. What has been so powerful with my daughter is that she has enabled me to experience a different form of love and appreciate it in a way I've never experienced before. That love has grown just as she has. But even when she was a baby, I experienced what it was to share unconditional love with someone for the first time in my life. India's approach to life reminds me of how I want to show up to the world – fearless, and determined to get the most out of each day.

Even if you don't have children yourself, the younger generations have the power to teach us so much about the world. It might be just reminding us of how we also used to live life with joy, curiosity, and an open appreciation of the small things that, as adults, we often overlook. As time passes, we can lose some of those qualities due to our experiences causing us to become jaded about the world or numbing us to it. But that viewpoint can be recaptured and nurtured by spending valuable time with the children in our lives, and allowing them to be our teachers.

Lesson 67: You are Never Too Young to Make an Impact on the World

Too often we assume that it is the older generations who have all the answers – that their age is an indicator of their wisdom – but I don't think that's always the case. Inspiration can come from anyone at any age, and I think we are often held back by the assumption that we're too young to do something.

As mentioned in the previous chapter, I thought I was too young to become a dad. I also believed that I didn't have the necessary experience to take certain steps in my career when I was younger. But, after becoming a father, I learned so many lessons from my daughter – even when she was still a baby and couldn't even speak. She continues to make an impact in my world and inspires me every day. Eventually I realized that not only was I succeeding at being a dad, I was also becoming a better, fuller version of myself that I never would have been if I'd waited until I was 'ready' to take that step.

We should never put limits on ourselves because of our age. Greta Thunberg is a great example of this. The work she has done since she was a young teenager has highlighted and brought into the mainstream the import-ance of fighting climate change, not only for future generations but for the ones who are alive now. She has also shown young people that their voices count and should be heard. Whatever your views on her might be, you have to admire what she has achieved at such a young age and the bravery she has shown by standing up to some of the most influential people in the world.

We have a lack of progressive leaders at the moment, and we should be inspiring younger people to step forward into those roles. Too many young people are being led astray. Perhaps if they had younger leaders to look up to, there wouldn't be the same level of disconnection with the leadership of the country. The older leaders also don't seem to be making the right decisions. How can we expect long-term policies from people who might not live to see the benefits? We need selfless acts of leadership that make the best decisions for long-term gain rather than short-term popularity.

As parents, aunts, uncles, grandparents, caregivers, teachers or role models, we must empower the children within our care to believe that anything is possible, even at a young age. Any other mindset could create limitations. They are never too young to think about the impact they want to have on the world, and if they are genuinely passionate about something, they should just go for it.

I've never pushed my daughter into running, but she has naturally started to enjoy it. Recently, I wanted to see if she could run a kilometre with me, so we put on our trainers and went to the park. I went into it anticipating that she would probably run ten paces and then need to stop to catch her breath, and we would go home. But she set off in front of me and started running at a fast pace. When she eventually stopped to catch her breath, she did it for only a few seconds and then set off again. When we hit our target of a kilometre, she wanted to keep on running, but I told her we would build up to longer distances. Witnessing her dedication was really inspiring, and I came away from it incredibly proud of her. I am optimistic about India's future and what she could achieve with that mindset. My biggest goal in life is to nurture her to chase her dreams, because if she does, the things she achieves could be monumental.

We are currently raising the next generation of leaders. One of the greatest things we can do for them is to remind them that they are never too young to explore their full potential and the impact they can have on the world.

Lesson 68: Go Further Together

It was day one of the ultra-marathon in Sri Lanka, and only 30 miles in I was ready to give up. Hours ago, I'd lost the rest of the group, who were scattered either miles ahead of me or behind, and I was running alone. The heat was so intense that even a slow jog had raised my heart rate to 170 bpm, and it stubbornly refused to return to a lower level. I was damned if I ran and damned if I didn't. Running would raise my heart rate even higher, but walking meant more time in the sun. Giving up wasn't an option, as it wasn't as if I could just hail a taxi to take me to a hotel. I was in the middle of the Sri Lankan countryside with no way of contacting or alerting anyone to my situation. As quitting was off the table, I decided to sit down by the side of the path and rest for a few minutes to try to coax my heartbeat to return to something approaching its normal level.

Near-delirious from the toll the day had taken on me, I caught a slow movement in the corner of my eye. Only a few metres from me was a squirrel. The more lucid part of my mind questioned whether they had grey squirrels in Sri Lanka. As this thought circulated, the squirrel began to morph into another animal – a crocodile. I jumped up and sped away. Adrenaline pumped through me, a blast of energy that came from nowhere as I ran for my life. So many times, the race leaders had warned us about the risks of crocodiles and snakes. In my exhaustion, I'd sat down next to a crocodile – and hallucinated that it was a squirrel. When I finally slowed down, the shock of such a near-miss hit me, and all I could say was 'Fuck!' over and over again. I was even more dehydrated and now questioning my sanity. I had no other option but to continue my slow jog for the rest of the day and didn't sit down again.

By the time I finally finished that first day and returned to base camp, I didn't think I'd be able to go back out there for day two, but then I sat down to eat a simple meal with people who had been through what I had. We exchanged stories. One guy had nearly passed out; another had seen someone airlifted to hospital. We consoled each other and laughed about our struggles, and it helped to know I wasn't alone. Even though we could have backed out now that we were back at camp, where there was a driver to help us leave the race, none of us did so because we had a shared experience and were all in this together. We set off the next day to cover 56 kilometres knowing the pain that lay ahead for us, but now we had a collective goal and we wanted each other to succeed at what we'd set out to do.

Eleven months later, when I set out to start the 76 Marathons, I held this lesson close and made it part of our ethos: you go further together. With all my previous UK challenges, I'd had to do most of them with just a small team for company – or, when it came to the patio challenges, by myself. Either no one else could join me as we were in lockdown, or I was running on isolated routes, or I was completing the challenge in a wheel-chair. With the 76 Marathons, I wanted people to be able to run with me anywhere in the country – a sort of mobile, open house that anyone was welcome to drop in on. It was never about personal bests, people slowing others down or a sense of competition. It was instead about how far we could go together. Whenever anyone showed up at the start line to run with us, I was so grate-ful they were there to support me, and I wanted to learn how our run would support them in return. Seeing strangers come together and achieve something so sig-nificant was inspiring. It wasn't about running as quickly as we could but rather finishing together.

Fundamentally, going further together is about collab-oration. Whether that means joining up with a stranger to run for a couple of hours or spending time supporting those who others might see as competitors. It applies to every industry, profession and interest. We have the choice to view others in a similar field as either our future collaborators or our current competitors.

I think a mindset where we view everyone as a com-petitor comes from a place of inadequacy. We believe there is not enough room to accommodate everyone, and deep down, we may even feel our abilities are insuf-ficient for us to carve out a place for ourselves. When we are reluctant to share our space or are protective of what we do, it ultimately comes from a negative place where our world remains small as we struggle to control everything within a rigid sphere. This damages our potential, and makes it feel like we have either won or lost opportunities in life, rather than gaining something from every experience.

When we approach things with a mindset of plentifulness, we feel secure in ourselves and our place in the world. We see more opportunities, and we *have* more opportunities because we are willing to help others on their journey and, in turn, accept help. I don't do these challenges because I think I'm better than anyone else. I do them because they fulfil me, help others, and foster incredible connections between people. The more people I share them with, the better.

Lesson 69:
There is Room for All of Us

I was in the middle of a challenge when a reporter approached me. Expecting the usual questions about the toll it was having on my physical and mental health, I was confused when they asked if I felt threatened by someone else who was also setting themselves extreme challenges. They wanted to know whether I was concerned that the individual would take the spotlight from me. My mind went blank, as this wasn't something that had ever crossed my mind.

When people talk about the spotlight or your 'appeal', it shifts the focus onto the question of ego, validation and potentially narcissism. The challenge space shouldn't be about that, and I don't think it is most of the time. Ultimately, if you're concerned about other people drawing attention away from you, it indicates a fear of how fragile your world is. There is insecurity at play because you probably don't believe you are enough to hold people's attention or survive without it. If you believe in what you are doing and find it fulfilling, whether people know about it or are interested in it should be irrelevant. Although those in the challenge space might do similar things on paper, we are all completely different. So many factors make each of us unique, such as how we articulate ourselves, our Why, our approach to our challenges, and the team dynamic. These factors enable us to differentiate ourselves from each other. There's no one type of challenge, so we don't all attract one type of audience. Our appeal is broad and varied.

So, when it came to the reporter who was asking me if I was worried about someone else taking the spotlight from me, I only had one answer. It was that I didn't even think about the spotlight, let alone worry about it. If anything, I want more people to feel inspired by what I do so many more people can discover the benefits of running and other physical activities. If we're going to spread that message, we need as varied a group as possible in the challenge space who will appeal to a wide demographic.

What a dull world it would be if there weren't others daring to dream. But what sort of message are we passing on if *we* are allowed to dream but feel threatened by anyone else with the same or a similar dream? It is a much healthier dynamic to welcome everyone. Our shared interests can break down any barriers that may have previously held us apart. I am so proud to be a part of the challenge community and to watch how many people within it support each other – and long may it continue. Because the reality is that, at some point, my body probably won't be able to continue with these feats of endurance, and my time will come to an end. Instead of waiting until that happens to pass the baton on, I want to pass it on now and support all those entering this space. There is certainly room for more of us, because there are still more people we can reach.

I have made a point of highlighting the other incredible challenges that people are taking on by starting a podcast where I interview some of the most inspiring people pushing themselves in new and exciting ways. For one of the episodes, I spoke with Sean Conway, who is someone I really admire. His recent achievement of 105 consecutive Ironmans makes him one of our arena's most remarkable individuals. An Ironman is a triathlon where you swim 2.4 miles, cycle for 112 miles, and then run a marathon. Sean did this every single day for 102 days with no rest days in between, beating the previous world record of 101. At this point, he should have been on the front page of every newspaper in the country. But even more impressively, he kept going and decided to let fate choose how many more Ironmans he would complete. Each day, he would toss a coin, which would determine whether he would do another Ironman the following day. At the end of day 105, the result of the coin toss meant that he would stop, and he held himself to that.

Wherever you find fulfilment, I hope you are greeted with the attitude that there is room for everyone. And if there isn't, that there is the chance to cultivate one. I'm not naive. I know that not everyone will encounter the welcome they deserve. There will be others who operate from a place of insecurity and try to prevent your progression. What this says about them is that they are not secure in themselves, rather than being a reflection of what you are trying to achieve.

We still have the choice of being a maverick and striving to enter any area with head held high, creating room for everyone. We can then leave the door wide open, so others can follow. We can even help them take the first steps through that door by guiding, mentoring and supporting them. When we take that approach, we can create something truly extraordinary.

Lesson 70: Don't Rely on Validation from Others

When we start something new, we need to do it with our heads held high, as this pride in ourselves sets the tone of the journey. There will always be setbacks, low points, and times when we feel discouraged. But if we believe in what we are doing and our right to attempt it, we have already won a large part of the battle.

Persistence and self-belief are essential. If I had listened to every person who tried to discourage me from doing something, or accepted every door slammed in my face, I would have given up years ago. We have to grow a protective barrier around ourselves and try not to let these things pierce through it. I now rarely care what people say about me, because I know that paying attention to it is unproductive at best and potentially catastrophic at worst.

Instead, I utilize the rejections and hurdles I face to spur me on. We are often advised not to hold on to negative energy, but I don't entirely believe in that. Doubt or rejection from others can be used in a constructive way too. In the depths of any challenge, when things are tough, I reflect on the people who have done me wrong and the rejections I have faced. It is just a way to use that negative emotion for something positive. I find it can be a powerful reserve to draw on when things look bleak and I'm wondering whether I'm going to complete something, or I'm doubting my reasons for even starting it. Knowing that I want to prove to myself and the doubters that I can do it keeps me going in those times. Some might consider that negative, but I honestly believe it is a *necessary* quality. Because too often, we can take rejection or a lack of support to heart, and give up.

When we have made some progress and secured a few wins, we have to be proud of our accomplishments. Many of us struggle in this modern world to acknowledge the work we have done. We seem to find it incredibly difficult to say nice things about ourselves. We can often recognize the achievements of others but struggle to apply the same criteria to ourselves. This partly comes down to the speed at which we live our fast-paced lives. There is little time for reflection or evaluation before we move on to the next thing. This becomes so embedded in our behaviour that it becomes part of our mindset. Five years pass by in a whirlwind of attainment but very little acknowledgement. The latest challenge or goal is all we focus on, with little emphasis on what came before.

This pattern can be broken, however, and I know this because I have done it myself. It begins with setting aside a little time after each achievement, big or small, to acknowledge the journey that led to the accomplishment. I have learned to reflect on each day of a challenge and what that single day will contribute to my overall success. I do this whether my achievements are acknowledged by anyone else or not.

Instead of waiting for someone else – such as your boss, colleague, partner or friend – to tell you that you've done a good job, you should just do it yourself. Remove the necessity for it to be acknowledged by others. Otherwise, when you finally achieve what you've set out to do, you might be surprised by the silence that you're met with. Sometimes, people are too busy with their own lives to pay attention to yours, or sometimes they ignore it intentionally for a variety of reasons. This doesn't mean that you have to tell all of these people that you're proud of yourself. This process of validation is internal.

If you rely on other people's praise for momentum or fulfilment, there is a good chance you will become disheartened. This is because you have no control over how people view what you're doing or their level of involvement. If you don't receive external recognition for what you do, it does not mean your work lacks value. You don't need outside input to validate your contributions. Instead, you can become your own champion by being proud of yourself and your accomplishments.

Lesson 71: Never Give Up

Four months after finishing the 76 Marathons, I was in Stanmore to support my friend, Jonny, on his ninth day of running the entire length of the London Underground. He had set himself the challenge of running all eleven tube lines in eleven days to raise money for charity. He was running between each station above-ground and tackling a different line each day. I had joined him for the Jubilee line run on day nine, which entailed 57 kilometres from Stanmore to Stratford. The rule was we had to run to each station and touch it before proceeding to the next one on the map.

In the days leading up to it, I had decided to only do a half marathon with Jonny. The most I had run since the 76 Marathons was 10 kilometres, as I had to give my injuries a chance to heal. I also hadn't done any training or preparation to attempt 57 kilometres in one day. On average, I only ran 4–5 kilometres each time I went out, so I was just there to support my friend and see how my body reacted to a 21k run.

An alarm at 5 a.m. woke me up so I could meet Jonny and his team at Stanmore underground station for our 6.30 a.m. start. Most of the UK was going through an unexpected heatwave, and we wanted to get as many kilometres as possible under our belts before the city heat began to impact us. Jonny had already run around 400 kilometres in the last week, so he was suffering from the consequences by the time I met up with him. He was in a lot of pain, and his body was seizing up, so his range of movement wasn't great. But he had a brilliant team of professionals running alongside him who were trying to patch him up along the way so he could keep running for the next three days.

That day, supporting Jonny became my Why. I could see that he was suffering and I knew that running with him would help him keep going. As the kilometres passed, I decided to try for the full 57 kilometres, as I couldn't imagine leaving him only a third of the way through. I was going to push on. It was not going to be easy, and definitely not something advised by my team, but I wanted to test myself and see if I still had the mental strength to continue going even when my mind was telling me to stop. The four months of rest since the 76 felt like a long time and I wanted to know if I could still do it.

Running between the stations, I managed to get lost three times, so I had to pick up my pace at times to try to catch up with Jonny and his team. Psychologically, it was a massive test for me, as although I could rely on muscle memory and my fitness levels, I hadn't put my body through anything like that for months.

The injuries I had from the 76 Marathons had been a setback, and I had found it difficult to see when or how

I would return to running extreme distances again. But I knew that I didn't ever want to use my setbacks as an excuse for halting my progression. By testing myself without any training or preparation, I discovered that my body could still cover a substantial distance in a day. It was also a testament to my strength and conditioning coach, Nick, as his work with me in the gym had kept my body in good shape.

I reached Stratford incredibly proud that I'd pushed myself to be there for my friend every step of the way. I was so relieved that I had allowed myself the time to heal over the four months leading up to that and for never giving up on challenging myself. The positive psychological impact that one day of running had on me was incredible. The weather was beautiful. I'd met an amazing group of runners and had some really interesting conversations about their lives and what they hoped to achieve with their own running. I felt so much gratitude for the life I was living and the opportunities I had even when I least expected it. I felt lucky to have been able to take the day off work to run with a friend, and that day had become so much more.

The following morning, I lifted a personal best in the gym, which shows how crucial our mindset is when pushing ourselves beyond what we thought was possible.

I felt as though I could begin considering a new challenge. The question was, what would it be?

Lesson 72: The Fears You Don't Face Will Become Your Limitations

We all tell ourselves stories about ourselves, and if we repeat them enough times, we start to believe them. These ideas of what we can't do or aren't suited to can quickly turn into fears, and unfaced fears create barriers around us. It can feel like those barriers are there to protect us from feeling awkward, embarrassed or out of our depth, but what they actually do is limit how we live our lives.

To move past these limitations, we have to be honest with ourselves about what scares us. I could easily write that my biggest fear is running in the heat and spend this chapter addressing that, but it wouldn't be truthful. Yes, running in the heat is something I've encountered that unsettles me, but it isn't one of my biggest fears. In fact, as I touched on earlier, my biggest fear is love. I've spent many years avoiding connecting with anyone on a romantic level because I'm afraid of being hurt, but I'm starting to realize that if I continue like this, I will miss out on a large part of what life has to offer. That fear of love will limit my life's experiences.

My parents' divorce showed me how love, and falling out of love, can rip a person or family apart; and ever since then, my view of love has never been particularly positive. Before India was born, it had only ever brought me pain. Consequently, I withdrew from making that type of connection to protect myself and ensure it wouldn't impact me again. But then, one day, I became a father to a little girl. It was not immediate love, as I wasn't even sure how I felt in the early days, but having a daughter broke down my barriers one by one. I had always viewed love through a particular lens, but how I felt about India was different, and it showed me that love comes in many forms. Had my daughter not come into this world, I may never have experienced this. It changed so much for me. There is still a long way for me to go, but it was a huge step in shifting my perspective on love.

I've been so blessed with the life that I've had, but the biggest turning point for me was when India came into the world. It opened me up to the idea of facing my fear of meeting someone and letting them in. Weddings are emotional, and in the right circumstances and with the right people they can trigger even the toughest person. Witnessing the power of love has shown me why it's worth taking the risk. I've come to realize that my experience of love is only one side of it, and over the past few years I have been able to see what makes it so special. My biggest fear is of being hurt, but I can see now that when you meet the right person, you will have someone by your side who tests you, supports you, and inspires you to be the best version of yourself. Being a part of that brings fulfilment of a different kind. The fear of love is still deep within me, but the older I get, the more open I am to facing it.

What I am certain of is that the fears we don't face will become our limitations. If we don't test them or find ways to work around them, our lives will forever be restricted by them.

Facing our fears takes a bit of soul-searching, as we first have to admit to ourselves what we are most afraid of. Once we can name it, we can begin to address it, to ensure it doesn't hold us back. The more we build something up in our heads, the bigger the limitation becomes. We then have a choice. Do we live with that emotion and restriction for the rest of our lives? Or do we face it head-on? I am certain that the fulfilment we find after facing our fears head-on makes the decision an easy one.

Lesson 73: Never Stop Learning

The other morning, I woke up to the sound of cups and plates being moved around. One of India's favourite games is to have a teddy bear's picnic on the dining room table, so I presumed that it was her setting up for the game. After a couple of minutes, the clunking noise continued, and it was clear it was time to investigate. I wandered into the kitchen, and India was holding out a glass for me. She proudly showed me the empty dishwasher and explained that she had unpacked it all herself and was about to bring me a glass of water. I was so impressed by her initiative. For weeks, I had been showing her how to unload the dishwasher, and she had spontaneously decided to give it a go by herself. She didn't need me to show her again because she had taken another step towards independence.

It is amazing how she is constantly learning – picking up new words and new skills. As we get older we lose touch with a child's curiosity and desire to learn, but there is always more to learn wherever we are in life, as we are never the finished article. Seeing India learn and grow each day has been a big wake-up call for me and reminds me that we need to keep asking questions and trying new things, because there is so much more for us to gain. Everyone is a work in progress.

India has inspired me to be curious about every aspect of my life – at home, with friends and at work. When I first started working with my nutritionist, Renee, she asked me how I like to work. I told her that with every team member who joins me, it's important for me to be able to learn as much from them as possible. I don't just want to be told what the answer is; I need to know the reasoning behind it. It turned out that working with Renee, with her unique skills and expertise, would be a pivotal aspect of my challenges.

Not only does this approach make me less reliant on other people, it also gives me a deeper understanding so I can make my own informed decisions in the future. Being able to make quick decisions can make or break a challenge, and I don't want my lack of knowledge to be the deciding factor in whether I succeed.

Just like India, when we learn how to do things ourselves, we become more independent and able to make our own decisions. What a freeing feeling that is.

Lesson 74: Create a Ripple

Every interaction we have has the potential to create a ripple. When we help others without expecting anything in return, or inspire someone to find fulfilment or pursue their dreams, this has a positive impact on their lives and, in turn, their positive actions can go on to inspire others. The more you do, the more ripples you create, and the more positivity comes out of it.

I have seen this ripple effect in action in my own work. At the start of the 76 Marathons challenge, only one person was running with us, and by the end, there were hundreds. What will they go on to do to help others? When I was running marathons around my patio in lockdown, I had a call with ten students who went on to do their own patio challenges. Who will they connect with and inspire? When I mentor people with their own challenges, I always want to learn about their Why as I know it will inform the success of their work. Who will they share their own unique way of finding fulfilment with?

We each have the potential to connect with thousands if not hundreds of thousands of lives. And if even only a handful of them go on to help or inspire others, we are reaching a point of substantial change. This ripple effect is now what I focus on when I create anything, because it is a powerful change-maker and can spread outwards around the world – and through generations.

People have the power to create harmful ripples too, and sometimes the most positive thing we can do is to prevent that negativity from going any further. One of the most powerful days from the 76 challenge was when I was joined by an inspirational young woman who had lost her sister to suicide just three weeks prior. The circumstances that led up to her sister's death were unimaginably traumatic and she could so easily have been consumed by anger – the start of the ripple – and yet she wanted to break the cycle and run with us in her sister's honour that day to raise awareness and spread a positive message that help is out there. Running had been her sister's support mechanism for so long, so she wanted to run in her footsteps and show support for the Samaritans, who had given her a lifeline. I was so moved by her story because she epitomized everything that I was running for and, despite having never run one before, she ran the whole marathon with us that day. She showed me that we can change the narrative and turn a negative ripple into a positive one.

Remarkable achievements also shift people's perception of what is possible, even when the person providing that inspiration faces something others might view as a limitation. Just like people rarely focus on my anxiety, people rarely focus on Tano's way of walking. Instead, they see a man who beat the odds to walk again. Tano has used this to help people with spinal injuries, and he will drive hundreds of miles to visit them in hospitals as he knows how crucial those first few months are. He shows them what might be possible and that they have their whole lives to prove the odds wrong. It might be a million to one, but if there's still a one, then there's still a chance.

When we witness people who have faced challenges that we haven't and how they react to the world in a positive way, we can adopt their approach to life ourselves. Because if they can do it, why can't we? If Tano can learn to walk again, he can inspire someone to learn to run.

Too often, we look at ourselves and assume we can't make any difference to the world as just one person. It can lead to us deciding not to participate or giving up trying to create change. In reality, the decisions we make when it comes to how we present ourselves to the world and finding something to motivate us have a huge impact. Even if we choose to simply find something to fulfil us and combine this with a positive approach to life, we will go through life with purpose. At least one life will benefit. People might also look at us and find inspiration in what we are doing – the happiness that fulfilment has brought to our lives – and decide to emulate this themselves. A positive outlook multiplied can become a norm. Barriers are removed, and setbacks are viewed as valuable lessons.

I find this idea of creating a ripple hugely motivational, because it means we aren't just trying to achieve our goals for personal reasons, we are doing it for other people too. We are doing it for the example it will set and how it makes others feel, so that another ripple can begin.

Lesson 75: Give Someone a Reason to Live

The reason I feel so passionately about giving other people a reason to live is because in my early twenties I almost lost my battle with depression and, in turn, my life. In that make-or-break moment I paused, and that pause saved my life. Why did I hesitate? I felt I had no reason to live and yet I did not follow through. Even if the reason was not clear to me at the time, something was clearly worth living for. From that day on, I committed myself to finding out what that was.

That young man had given up on his future. He could not imagine the joy and fulfilment to come. He could not believe that, one day, he would have a beautiful daughter who makes every day worthwhile and that he would be a father she is proud of. He could not see himself crossing the finishing line, running miles for charity, meeting people from all over the world who share his passion, achieving the previously unachievable, starting a successful company that is a leader in its field, or finding fulfilment and purpose through helping others. None of that was apparent to him. How could it be? When you fast-forward to what my life has become, who could have written that story? And none of it would have happened if I had taken my life that day.

So if there's even the slightest chance that someone might not go on to experience what their future holds for them, we have to try to give them a reason to live. No one should have a lifetime taken from them. Because who knows what their future will hold? They could be a friend, parent, colleague, future inspirer, leader, innovator or any manner of person. It is truly inspirational when we consider all the possibilities stretched out in front of us. The paths that will intertwine, the future friendships, relationships and ventures. We cannot underestimate what the future has in store for us. One experience or achievement leads to another, sometimes heading off in unimagined or anticipated directions.

What I am doing right now with my life won't necessarily connect with everyone, but I hope that the positivity and energy I put out into the world will have an impact on someone, who will in turn impact positively on someone else and so on, so that people feel less alone. Ultimately, I am striving for every person who is born into this world to feel more fulfilled. We all have the ability to contribute to that by showing people what is possible.

The key to this is finding your Why. There will always be highs and lows in the days, weeks and years of your life. But when you have found something that genuinely excites you, it will anchor you during stormy times. It will be a haven you can turn to while you wait for the hard times to pass by. There is always the chance of discovering new ways of finding fulfilment as well. One day, I won't be able to run these challenges anymore, and

I'll have to find something else to take their place to feel fulfilled. I have no idea what that will be right now, but I know that I will find it.

My uncle has always been known for being quite an emotionally reserved, quiet person – and, consequently, difficult to read. He surprised me recently at a family gathering when he asked if he could have a word with me. He told me that everyone is born to be great at something. But not everyone is lucky enough to discover what it is. He wanted me to know that he had been watching what I had been doing recently and it was clear that I had found what I was great at, which made him incredibly proud. It was a beautiful thing to be told, and everyone should have the chance to have those words spoken to them.

My uncle was right: everyone in the world is born to be great at something, and it's discovering what that greatness is that brings us hope. I was very lost in my early twenties, swamped by depression and consumed by the belief that my life had no meaning or purpose to it. Now, ten years later, I am writing a book on resilience. Not only that, on World Mental Health Day the prime minister awarded me the Points of Light award for my services around mental health.

Life likes to surprise us. Together, let's share all the endless ways in which it can, and spread this message of hope. I can't imagine any more significant achievement than someone telling us we are the reason they are still here today.

Lesson 76:
Fortune Favours the Brave

When I first found out that I was going to be a father, I was left feeling incredibly vulnerable and scared about what the future had in store for me. I didn't feel prepared to be a dad. I also feared the impact my previous mental health struggles would have on my child and that they might inherit them from me. Would my child have the same difficulties as me at school? Did I have the skills to help them through that if they did? All I could think about was not wanting my child to struggle in the ways that I had, and doubting that I could help them. This uncertainty about the future and doubt in my capabilities as a father carried on for months, and made me feel very isolated. I had fallen into the trap of concerning myself with what the future held. My anxiety spiralled and I felt consumed by worry as I didn't have any reassurance to anchor me.

When India was born, the reality of my responsibilities towards her was realized, and I continued to feel uneasy that I wouldn't be the dad she needed. A few days after she was born, a parcel arrived with my name on it, and I was surprised to see a man's solid metal bracelet inside. Running around the outside of it were the words 'Fortune Favours the Brave' with India's date of birth underneath. I remember sitting on our sofa holding that bracelet as I ran my thumb over the inscription. It was the reminder that I needed to be brave. And that by being brave, and by being consistent in my bravery, fortune would come from that.

Fortune looks different to everyone. My interpretation of fortune in that moment was to have a happy and healthy child. For that to happen, I would have to face my fears, embrace that feeling of vulnerability for as long as it lasted, and commit to doing the best I could. It was like someone had seen into my soul. After staring at the bracelet in disbelief and wondering who could have sent it, I put it on and resolved to face life head-on.

I never did find out who sent me that gift, but it changed my approach to life forever. Perhaps that is part of the beauty of the story – that it arrived exactly when I needed it.

I have carried those words into everything I do. When I look down at my wrist and read 'Fortune Favours the Brave', I know that whatever it is, if I bring my whole self I can face it and do it well. I know that's true because of the person India has become. When I look at her now, I am incredibly proud of how she has developed and the child she has grown into. I also know that I have played a massive part in her evolution. I was brave, and from that came my fortune.

At that time, my interpretation of 'fortune' was centred around India, but now she's older it changes

depending on what I am faced with. Once you understand what fortune means to you, you will know how
far you are willing to go to achieve it and how brave
you will have to be to get it.

Fortune doesn't have to be grand plans for multimillion-
pound businesses or expensive houses. Fortune can be
opening yourself up to love, reconnecting with someone
from your past, nurturing self-confidence, becoming
comfortable with your body, or being excited each morning by the day ahead. Bravery doesn't have to be dashing
into burning buildings or putting your life on the line. It
can be opening your heart even though it terrifies you,
reaching out to someone even though you fear rejection,
believing in yourself even when for years you have been
told you are not enough, learning to do the best for your
body even when you think it has let you down, or having
the strength to try different things until you find one that
brings you fulfilment.

Looking to the future, for me, fortune means peace. I
want to feel at peace because, at times, I can be unsettled
by my thoughts. By being brave and facing what life
throws at me, I know I will one day achieve this.

Words can change lives – those four words on that
unexpected gift certainly changed mine. That is why I
have written this book, in the hope that somewhere in
these pages there are words that will connect with you,
whether they provide a different perspective on what
might be a seemingly impossible situation, or inspire

you to find your Why to bring a newfound purpose to each day.

Move forward, take action, allow yourself to rest, find peace, find joy, whatever it is you need to make this life an enjoyable one. All of these things require bravery, but each one will bring you a fortune.

What Do You Want to Be Remembered For?

What do you want to be remembered for? This is the question that motivates me every single day. I don't just mean at the end of my life, either. Today is far more important than tomorrow. Today is guaranteed, and tomorrow is not. If we put off thinking about what we want to achieve with our lives, there is no guarantee that we will still be here to see it or have the good health we might need to make it happen. Why delay the things we want or hope to do in life? We can often focus too much on the future, as if it is owed to us – when, in reality, there are never any guarantees.

If, God forbid, something did happen to me tomorrow, I can honestly say I could lie on that hospital bed and know I have left a legacy my daughter can be proud of and look up to. But that doesn't mean I will give up on doing my best to create a better world for her. There is still more that I can add to my story, and I know this will include future challenges. I'm excited to see where the journey takes me.

For me, I want to live a life full of adventure, but the most important achievement of all is for my daughter to be proud of me and for my family to be proud of me too. Most of all, I want to leave this planet in a better place than I found it. To do any of these things, I have to take action. Because sometimes we are only one decision away from changing our own lives – and the lives of those around us.

Now it is your turn.

You have the ability to make a difference, so ask yourself: what do you want to be remembered for?

Acknowledgements

I would not be the person I am today, and nor would I have achieved the things I have, had I not had these special people in my life, inspiring and supporting me to push on and overcome any hurdle I have faced, both mentally and physically. You are the reason this book has to come to life.

India, my beautiful little girl, other than life itself, you're my greatest gift. The day you came into this world you changed my life and myself forever. The future is so exciting knowing I have you in it. This book highlights the things I have done, and those I can't wait to do with you. My proudest achievement is seeing you grow into the person you continue to be.

Thank you to my mum and dad for being patient with me. Having me as your son was never easy, and I have put you through so much, yet your belief and support in me has never dwindled. I'm not a conventional person, but I hope the things I have done, and continue to do, make you proud. Thank you for all the sacrifices you have made for me to get to where I am today.

My incredible sister, Georgia, the rock of this family. You make us all so proud; you have gone on to achieve things that no one in this family has done before. I don't think you know how special you are. You were put on this earth for a reason – you have gifts that can change this world and anyone you come into contact with.

Tano, Buki and Jack, the three of you have been through so much individually, and how you all have faced adversity is what inspires me the most about you. I admire the men you are, and the values you have. You have been there for me through the great times, and the tough ones too. You have played a huge part in shaping the man I am today.

My incredible team who have invested so much into me, believed in me when others did not, picked me up when I was down, and patched me back together when I was broken, there is nothing on earth that's worth more than you all. We have achieved things no human on earth has done before, we have pushed the boundaries of what's possible, and we have enabled people to believe in the unbelievable. There are 76 chapters in this book, but this story is far from finished. Reece, Chris, Charlie, Simon, Nick, Ben, Renee, Sharon, Megan, Kris, George, Tom, Lynsey, Hannah, Kenty, Tufnell, Jamie and Sam, THANK YOU!

Shirley, my therapist, you have helped me face my biggest battle of all: my mental health. Without you I truthfully don't know if I would be here today. Your kindness, empathy and ability to shine a light when it was needed the most has helped me more than you know. You have been one of my greatest supports in life; I feel optimism now when faced with any hurdle; I feel at peace knowing I have you in my life.

Charlotte and Megan, the industry I find myself in can be harsh and unfair, and it feels at times like if it had its way I would not have a place in it. You have picked me up every time it knocks me down; you believe in me and remind me why it's important to keep going. Without you both the world wouldn't know half the things I've done. Thank you for not giving up on me.

To Amy M, Amy W and everyone at Penguin, thank you for believing in me enough to make this book become a reality. I needed your belief to have the courage to do this. I've strayed away from doing this for so long out of fear, and I'm so grateful that now I have. Out of all the people in this world to work with on this, I'm so happy it was you two.

Lastly I want to thank my younger self. Life threw you many curve balls, some out of your control, some self-inflicted. I want to thank you for having the courage to not follow through when you were at your lowest and ending your life that day. Because of that moment I was able to grow, to find peace, to help others who have struggled to process things the way I have been lucky enough to; to travel the world and see its beauty, and the people within it; to fall in love, and become a father; to start a business, and test the boundaries of what's possible. I want you to know how grateful I am, and know I intend making the most of every single ounce of myself so I can give people the life they deserve – like the life you gave me.

My life is far from over, and it's inevitable I will be faced with more struggles and challenges, but knowing I have you all by my side, anything can be overcome.